The Complete Guide to Whiplash

Michael R. Melton

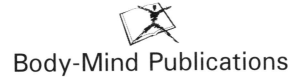

Body-Mind Publications

7631 Forest Park Dr NW
Olympia, WA 98502
(800) 295-3346
(360) 866-0537
Fax (360) 866-0537
bodymind@olywa.net
www.bodymindonline.com

The Complete Guide to Whiplash

By Michael R. Melton

For information about other related materials, including our monthly newsletter
the *Soft-Tissue Review,* please contact:

Body-Mind Publications
7631 Forest Park Dr NW
Olympia, WA 98506
(800) 295-3346
(360) 866-0537

Library of Congress Catalog Card Number: 98-96767
ISBN 0-9668091-0-6
First paperback edition published 1998.

Contents

A special thanks to Alissa Zwanger, for the cover design and for her invaluable
assistance in editing and proofing.

Introduction

"According to an estimate of the National Safety Council, there were 11,900,000 motor vehicle accidents in the United States in 1993. Of these, 2,750,000 were rear-end collisions. Although the precise number of whiplash injuries per year cannot be determined, a rather rough estimate is more than one million."[37]

Whiplash is a modern problem. While head and neck injuries certainly occurred before the invention of modern transportation, they were mostly limited to falls and the injuries of war. It was not until the invention of the train—not the automobile—that these types of injuries became common to the general population.

Train travel in the 19th century was a hazardous and potentially lethal activity. Train schedules virtually random, telegraphs had yet to be invented and so there was no way to communicate problems on the line, and in many parts of the eastern U.S there did not even exist a standard time between different cities by which to coordinate schedules. The result was hundreds of railroad crashes. Exacerbating the problem was the fact that railway cars were flimsy, wooden structures with no protection for the occupants. Railway collisions were a common occurrence.

Soon, a group of people started coming forward who claimed that they had been injured in train crashes, but had no obvious evidence of injury. The railroads, at the time run by men seeking quick profit, rejected these claims as faked.

Some physicians, however, took the injuries seriously. In 1882, the British surgeon Dr. John Eric Erichsen authored the book *Concussion of the Spine*.[388] In it, he wrote,

"It must, however, be evident to you all, that in no ordinary accidents can the shock, physical and mental, be so great as in those that occur on railways. The rapidity of the movement, the momentum of the persons injured and of the vehicle that carries them, the suddenness of its arrest, the helplessness of the sufferers, and the natural perturbation of mind that must disturb the bravest, are all circumstances which necessarily greatly increase the severity of the resulting injury to the nervous system, and which have led surgeons to consider these cases as somewhat exceptional and different from ordinary accidents."

Erichsen did not have access to MRI or CT scans. He couldn't study the effects of these injuries with electron microscopes or high-speed video cameras. Even with these limitations, he proved himself a brilliant observer and physician.

He was the first to recognize why these types of accidents cause injuries:

"I have often remarked that in railway accidents those passengers suffer most seriously from concussion of the nervous system who sit with their backs turned toward the end of the train which is struck. Thus when a train runs into an obstruction on the line, those who are sitting with their backs to the engine will probably suffer most; whilst if a train is run into from behind, those who are facing the engine will most frequently be the greatest sufferers. The explanation of this fact appears to me to be as follows. When a train runs into a stationary impediment, its momentum is suddenly arrested, whilst that of the passengers still continues. Those who are facing the engine are in the first instance thrown suddenly and violently forwards off their seats against the opposite side of the compartment; hence they will frequently be found to be cut about the head and face, and more especially across the knees and legs, by coming in contact with the edge of the opposite seats...Those, on the other hand, who are sitting with their backs to the engine, being carried backwards when the momentum of the carriage is suddenly arrested are struck at once; and if travelling rapidly, are jerked violently against the backs of their seats, and thus suffer in the first instance and by the first shock from concussion of the spine...The oscillations to which the body is subjected in these accidents are chiefly felt in those parts of the vertebral column that admit of most movement, viz., at the junction of the head and neck, of the neck and shoulders, and of the trunk and pelvis."

Seventy years before the first engineering tests had been performed on whiplash, Erichsen had correctly identified why whiplash injuries are more hazardous than other types of collisions, and had described the exact whiplash motion.

Erichsen admitted that he did not understand the biological mechanism behind such injuries, but, from his observations, termed these injuries "concussion of the spine." Other surgeons, hired by the railroads to fight injury claims, ridiculed the notion of railway injuries in general and spinal concussion in particular. Ironically, and 115 years later, some of the most recent literature on whiplash has found evidence that the spinal cord and the spinal nerves may indeed be traumatized, or "concussed," during whiplash movements.

The last few years have brought some of the most exciting developments in the understanding of whiplash. Careful research has started to show how the spine can be injured, even in low speed collisions. These new findings will help us not only understand how to help patients recover, but eventually help us avoid these injuries in the first place.

Understanding the complexity of the whiplash syndrome is the key to solving the problem. I hope that the information contained in this guide will increase the knowledge among professionals about whiplash, and expedite the day when this problem no longer exists.

Michael Melton

Chapter One

Biomechanics
No Vehicle Damage
Factors and Variables

Biomechanics

Nearly one third of all motor vehicle accidents are rear-end collisions,[37] and it is this type of accident that is responsible for most whiplash injuries. A solid understanding of the whiplash phenomena requires a basic knowledge of how the injury occurs. Biomechanics—the study of how mechanical forces affect living organisms—is useful in explaining how even a "minor" rear-end collision can result in a serious injury.

To illustrate the biomechanics of a common rear-end collision, let's use a simple two-car model. In this example, the front car is stopped at a traffic signal. Let's have the rear car move forward at about 10 m.p.h. The person in the front car is relaxed and unaware of the rear car.[134] (Figure 1.)

When the cars hit, the energy in the moving rear car is transferred to the front car, and the front car is moved forward. Newton's First Law of Motion states that, "An object continues either at rest or in a state of motion in a straight line unless it is acted upon by an external force."

Thus, the front car is moved forward by the external force of the rear car. The back of the car seat pushes the front occupant forward as well, but since the head is not contacting any portion of the seat, it remains stationary, resulting in backward motion of the head relative to the body.[134] (Figure 2.)

At some point, the front vehicle stops (either by braking or hitting some other object). At this point, the front occupant's body is thrown forward. If the occupant is not wearing a seatbelt, and the collision is at a high speed, he or she may hit the steering wheel or windshield. If the person is wearing a shoulder restraint, the head may be thrown forward with a simultaneous twisting motion, resulting in a greater risk of injury to the neck.[134] (Figure 3.)

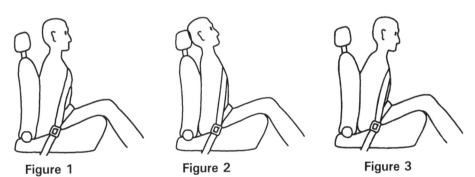

| Figure 1 | Figure 2 | Figure 3 |

In high speed collisions (over 10 m.p.h.), hyperextension, or the abrupt movement of the head backwards, usually causes the most damage since there are no anatomical restrictions to range of motion. As one study states, "neck extension is restrained only by the upper thorax, so that angulations of up to 120° may be attained, which are far beyond the physiologic maximum of 70°."[45]

Although hyperextension injuries generally do the most damage, hyperflexion or lateral flexion injuries do occur if the forces are severe enough.[21]

And the forces exerted on the neck and head during a rear-end collision can be very high:

"One G is the force of acceleration due to the earth's gravity, or 32.2 ft/sec². A fighter pilot begins to gray out at 6G. One cannot raise the body or extremities against 8G. If a 200-pound man is subjected to 8G, this is a force of 8 x 200 or 1,600 pounds. If a car is hit in the rear and accelerated to a speed of 10.8 miles per hour within the span of 100 milliseconds, the car and the driver are accelerated to 5G. Ommaya and Hirsch determined the occupant in this situation would stand a 50-50 chance of sustaining a concussion." [111]

The high forces experienced during a collision have been borne out by experimental studies with test subjects. McConnell[289,290] reported occupant G forces as high as 15G in collisions of just 5 m.p.h. In this situation, the average human head (typically weighing around 10 pounds) turns into a 150 pound load on the cervical spine (15G x 10 pounds = 150 pound). MacNab[91] wrote, "In acceleration injuries, the force applied to the neck is roughly equivalent to the weight of the head multiplied by the speed that the head is moving." It is easy to see how mechanical damage can occur to the body from a relatively minor collision. Luo and Goldsmith[90] looked specifically at where the forces in flexion injuries were focused, and they found that discs in the lumbar region experience the highest pressure changes, especially those at L3-L4; and that, "the muscle strain in the cervical region is much greater than that in the abdomen...The splenius capitis is stretched more than 30% during flexion whiplash."

Older studies have used cadavers and animals to examine specific types of lesions after whiplash injury. Some of the findings include,

- "tearing of the sternocleidomastoid and longus colli muscles, retropharyngeal hematoma, intra esophageal hemorrhage, tearing of the cervical sympathetic chain, distruption of the anterior longitudinal ligament, disk disruption, and facet joint capsular tears" in primates subjected to whiplash conditions.[50]
- In human experimental studies, MRI has "demonstrated ruptures of the anterior longitudinal ligament, horizontal avulsion of the vertebral end plates, separation of the disk from the vertebral end plates, occult fractures of the anterior vertebral end plates, acute posterolateral cervical disk herniations, focal muscular injury of longus colli muscle, posterior interspinous ligament injury, and prevertebral fluid collections."[37]

No Vehicle Damage Accidents

Some critics of whiplash will go to great lengths to "prove" that whiplash injuries do not exist, especially in low speed collisions. One study[2] that has been very popular with accident reconstructionists and insurance claims adjusters measured the amount of force placed on the human head while subjects "participated by actively moving or by being passively jostled in 12 different events." The highest G forces obtained were from having the subject, "plop in a chair;" the forces were measured at 10.1 G. The experimenters did not measure the range of movement of the head, however, just the force, so it is unknown if the head was hyperextended. This did not keep the researchers from concluding that, "the accelerations appeared to be greater than those seen in the same parts of the body during some no-damage motor vehicle impacts...With no-damage accidents, one can reassure an accident victim who had otherwise been frightened by rumors of the horror and the mystery that sometimes follows the MVA 'whiplash' scenario."

An editorial[165] in the same journal states: "Those who complain of pain after a minor insult often are already suffering from a preexisting condition, and their discomfort could have been exacerbated temporarily by the impact. It behooves us to investigate further the causes of persistent physical pain, if it can exist at all without a psychological component."

These researchers ignored the fact that whiplash in the real world does not compare well with experimental subjects in a laboratory wearing helmets who are warned in advance that they are to be "jostled." Unfortunately for whiplash opponents, the study's methodology was seriously flawed. In fact, the researchers did not even study the same type of motion that is experienced during rear end test collisions or even the correct parameters to compare the two. In addition, Cholewicki et al[198] reported that even in collisions resulting in 3-10 Gs of force, cervical spine ligaments experienced stretching beyond normal physiological ranges of motion.

MacNab,[91] writing in 1964, had already made the distinction between whiplash and laboratory experiments of this sort. "If, as a result of an accident, the head accelerates in relation to the trunk — backward, forward, or sideways — injury to the neck may result. Because lesions produced in this way differ from those resulting from forced passive movements of the head, it seems worth while to differentiate them by the term *acceleration injuries of the neck*."

The myth that low speed collisions are safe was put to rest by Robbins.[324] He discussed the physics of acceleration, and provided the following equation:

$$a = \frac{V^2}{2s}$$

Where:
α = acceleration
V = velocity of impact
s = the crush distance

According to this equation, the less a car is damaged or crushed in a collision, the higher the acceleration of the struck vehicle and the greater the risk of injury. Robbins wrote,

> "…on a vehicle with a chassis, no serious visual deformation may occur even though it is subjected to relatively high speeds of impact. Classically, we see this in the case of pickup trucks or all-terrain vehicles that are traditionally fitted with a solid bumper-to-bumper chassis. Many of these types of vehicles are subjected to relatively severe impacts with little or no resulting damage to their bodies and bumpers. The classic whiplash injury associated with a great deal of litigation is most likely founded on the reasoning that if there was little or no vehicle damage, no injury can result. Motor vehicle bodies or bumper-to-bumper chassis offer little or no crushing effect on arresting obstacles when impacted; thus, relatively high G forces can be experienced by occupants when rear-ended, resulting in whiplash injury. The use of stiff motor vehicle bodies and chassis will also produce a spiked G force loading to occupants, even if little damage occurs to vehicle body or chassis." [324]

Figure 4 shows the relationship between crush distance and G forces, and as we can see from this chart, vehicles that do not crush can experience very large accelerations at low speeds.

Whiplash not comparable to "plopping in a chair."

There is no relationship between vehicle damage and injury.

G Forces and Corresponding Injury that is Possible

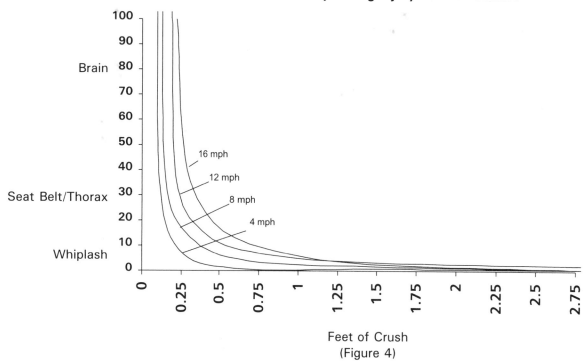

Feet of Crush
(Figure 4)

Engineering test collisions consistently show that the peak vehicle G forces in a collision are approximately twice as high as the average G forces. Furthermore, peak *occupant* G forces are about twice as large as peak *vehicle* forces. Thus, an occupant in a low speed collision with no damage to the vehicle may be at a significantly higher risk of injury than an occupant in a collision with a damaged vehicle. (For a more detailed discussion of this topic, please see our book *Low Velocity Whiplash Biomechanics*, available at (800) 295-3346.)

Furthermore, a study by Ono et al[300] found that even in collisions of just 5-mph, test occupants experienced cervical neck motions that were, "non-physiological motion of the vertebral segments."

Brault et al[187] in 1998 found in their test collisions that 29% of healthy subjects reported short-term symptoms from collisions of just 2.5 m.p.h.

How the Cervical Spine is Injured in Low Speed Collisions

A new set of studies have been published in the last year or two that are going to dramatically change the way we look at low speed collisions.

Since whiplash was first investigated in the 1950s, researchers have looked only at the external motions of the body during impact. Because these engineers saw no evidence of hyperextension, they naturally assumed that there was nothing happening during such crashes, and that injury was not possible. The latest literature, though, has started to take advantage of new technologies and has begun to look inside the body and to study the specific motion of each individual vertebra during rear end impact.

Facet Joint Injury

Injury to the cervical zygapophysial facet joints (from here on referred to as simply "facet joints" and highlighted in Figure 5) of the cervical spine has been documented in a number of studies over the last few years. Three recent studies in particu-

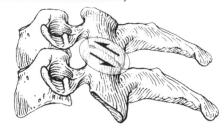

Figure 5

lar have looked at the role of facet joints in causing whiplash pain.

Fukui[220] determined the distribution of referred pain from the cervical facet joints by injecting the facet joint or by electrical stimulation of the nerves that supply the facet joints. From these tests performed on 61 patients, the following patterns were found. These areas of referred pain are very similar to the distribution of pain experienced by patients with whiplash-type injuries. (See Figure 6.)

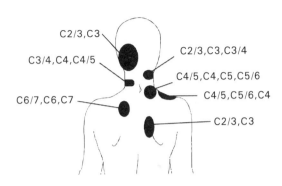

C2/3,C3
C3/4,C4,C4/5
C6/7,C6,C7
C2/3,C3,C3/4
C4/5,C4,C5,C5/6
C4/5,C5/6,C4
C2/3,C3

Figure 6

Another group of researchers performed the other two studies. In 1996, Lord et al[269] injected the medical branches of the dorsal rami in patients with whiplash-related pain. These are the nerves that innervate the facet joints of the spine. The authors found that 60% of the patients had evidence of facet joint injury. In another study, Lord et al[271] performed radio-frequency neurotomy on the same nerves of another group of whiplash patients. Although the long-term outcome was poor, 7 of 12 patients (58%) reported a relief of symptoms for a few months.

60% of whiplash patients show evidence of facet joint injury.

Thus, from these studies and others, we see that there is some kind of relationship between the whiplash injury mechanism and damage to the facet joints of the cervical spine. The problem to date has been identifying what mechanism in the whiplash motion is responsible for this damage, especially in low speed collisions.

Mechanism of Injury

An engineering study by Yang et al[372] provides some fresh insights. The authors focused on one aspect of the biomechanics of whiplash that is often overlooked—the fact that the cervical spine is subjected to a compressive force during the collision. This takes place at about 120 milliseconds into the impact, which also happens to be the approximate time that the head begins its movement backwards toward the head restraint—the time when shear forces are acting upon the lower cervical spine.

Yang et al[372] explained:

> "It is hypothesized that this axial compression, together with the shear force, are responsible for the higher observed frequency of neck injuries in rear end impacts versus frontal impacts of comparable severity. The axial compression first causes loosening of cervical ligaments making it easier for shear type soft tissue injuries to occur."

The following illustrations help illustrate this theory. During this particular phase of the impact, the cervical spine is subjected to a compressive force (Figure 7), while individual facet joints are subjected to shear forces (Figure 8). Shear forces are those caused by two bodies sliding in opposite directions from each other. In the following example, vertebrae C5 is moving backward with the upper part of the spine and head, while vertebrae C6 is moving forward with the torso.

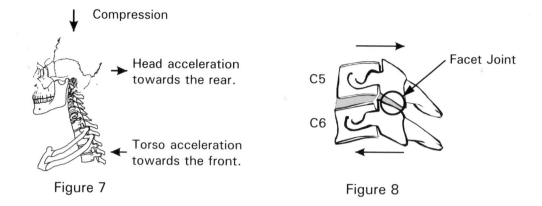

Figure 7

Figure 8

The researchers tested this theory by performing experiments on cadaver spine specimens. The specimens were subjected to compression, and then tested for shear resistance. The study found that the stiffness of the cervical spine decreased dramatically when a load was placed on the spine axially. The following table compares the difference in stiffness between a spine with no load and one with a load of 40 pounds.

Shear Stiffness (in N/mm)

	C2/C3	C3/C4	C4/C5	C5/C6
No Load	14.9	9.0	10.9	18.6
40 lbs Load	7.5	4.5	6.3	5.0
% Decrease in Stiffness	50%	50%	42%	73%

From this study we see that stiffness values, or the resistance to shear forces, can decrease as much as 73% when an axial load is placed on the spine. A load of 40 pounds may seem large, but it really isn't. As the researchers state:

"Although the vertical acceleration may seem small, it plays a significant role in the cervical spine biomechanics. The head generally possesses about 4.5 kg (10 lbs) of inertial mass. Even a small acceleration could generate a significant compressive force at the neck."

Thus, a 4g force on the head would result in a 40-pound compressive load. The exact amount of compression that the cervical spine experiences during impact has not been carefully measured in most studies. However, McConnell et al[289] reported that compressive G forces ranged from 1.0g to 1.5g in collisions at just 4-5 m.p.h. When adding the weight of the head already exerting a 10 lb force, this very low speed collision could result in possible loads of 20-25 lbs.

The final pieces of the puzzle have been put together by other researchers. Grauer et al[232] found that, when studying the effects of impact on cadaver spines, the spine does not bend smoothly as it does during controlled, normal extension of the neck. They found that the spine forms an S-shaped curve during the early phases of the impact—50-75 milliseconds. This S-shaped curve is caused by early flexion of the upper cervical spine at the same time that the lower cervical spine is undergoing extension.

Ono et al[300] independently confirmed this finding a few months later by studying high speed x-ray video of test subject cervical spines during low speed collisions. They found the following sequence of events:

1. Normal head position before impact.
2. Immediately after the impact, the car seat pushes the torso forward while the head remains stationary due to inertia. This results in a straightening of the spine and

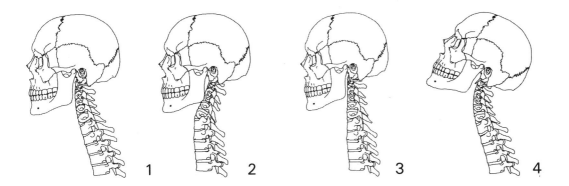

Figure 9

compresses the facet joints. As we saw above, this results in a weakening of the joints.

3. The S-shaped curve occurs in the spine at around 75 milliseconds, resulting in sharp bending of the lower spinal segments.
4. After the sharp bending occurs, the spine finally fully extends. Historically, this is the point where most scientists thought that injury was occurring—during the extension phase. According to the latest literature, the injury may have occurred before the head even reaches this point in the whiplash motion.

Whiplash motion is not normal head motion.

Researchers have determined that these motions of the cervical spine are not normal motion, and that the facet joints could potentially be injured during collisions that cause such neck movement.

Most interesting was the finding that this abnormal motion occurs in the region of C4-C6—the same segment of the spine where most whiplash lesions are found. (For further information on the types of injury that can occur, please see the section on Neck Pain.)

Factors and Variables

Accurately determining the forces present in a particular collision is impossible, because so many different variables are involved. Each crash possesses its own characteristics that can make the difference between an accident with no injury and an accident with serious injury. An accurate assessment of the actual forces from a collision requires the skills of an expert engineer. The potential risk of injury, however, can be roughly estimated by examining the following variables:

1. **The angle of the collision.** Was the patient's car hit straight on, from the side, or at some angle? The angle of collision will play a large role in determining what forces were placed upon the neck and head, and what tissues were damaged from these forces. A straight-on impact will generally be less hazardous than a collision from an angle, as the spine may be twisted in off-center impact. Because of their complexity, engineers have not yet performed tests on offset collisions.
2. **The speed and size of the rear car.** Obviously, the faster and heavier the rear car is moving, the more severe the forces placed on the occupant in the front car. A large truck going 5 mph can do much more damage than a small car going 20 mph.[90]
3. **The speed and size of the front car.** Also, if the front car is large, there may be less damage, but a small car can experience much higher accelerations in a minor impact.[21,45,90]
4. **Road conditions.** Was the road dry, wet, or icy? Was the road surface asphalt or gravel? Again, as in #3, the amount the car moves after the collision is critical, and the road surface can make a "minor" accident more severe than it at first appears.[21]
5. **Occupant head position.** Was the patient looking straight forward? Or was his head turned? A turned head will expose the spine to more complex stresses, resulting in a increased risk of injury.[21,137,168]

6. **Gender.** Research has consistently shown that women are at a much higher risk of developing chronic whiplash pain than are men. Experts have suggested that this increased risk may be due to differences in anatomy or seating position.

7. **Occupant awareness.** It is generally believed that whiplash trauma is less when the occupant has an opportunity to "brace" herself in the collision, preventing the head from being hyperextended. Bracing of the arms and legs, however, can result in trauma to these areas of the body. A clear picture of what the patient did the instant of the collision is imperative, although difficult to ascertain.[21,37] Sturzenegger et al[137] found that a surprised victim predicted worse injuries.

8. **Head restraints.** Most people mistakenly believe that the head restraint is a head "rest," and use it to rest their heads. The restraint should be positioned so that the back of the head touches it. Many adjustable head rests are set too low, so that they act as pivots during hyperextension, causing more injury. One study by Viano et al[353] found that only 10% of head restraints on the road are adjusted correctly. Another common problem is that seats in cars are set back at an angle, and many people drive leaning forward. In this situation, the head can fully hyperextend, even with a head restraint.[37,133] (See Safety Devices.)

9. **Safety belts.** Shoulder belts are very effective at saving lives in auto accidents, but there is some evidence that they can actually cause more damage in a rear end collision.[3] Why? Because the body is held in place, causing the head to suffer worse hyperflexion. The cervical spine may also undergo a twisting motion from the head restraint, causing a more complex injury. Furthermore, considerable soft-tissue damage in the chest and shoulder can be caused by the force of the body against the shoulder belt.[21] (See Safety Devices.)

10. **Secondary collisions.** Did the patient's car hit another object? All forces, be they acceleration or deceleration, have an effect on the occupant of the vehicle. A relatively minor collision can be made much more complicated and hazardous if other impacts are involved.

11. **Direct body impact.** Whiplash pain can be accompanied by minor or severe concussions if the head hits an object. Ask carefully as to whether any other parts of the body were injured in the collision.[38] If concussion did occur, patients may not remember due to mild amnesia.

12. **Loss of consciousness.** This can be important, as it indicates possible concussion or severe G forces in the injury. As we will see in the section on Brain Injury, however, concussion does not require loss of conciousness.

13. **Medical history.** A history of cervical spine degeneration, a history of headaches, or chronic soft-tissue pain can complicate the clinical picture.

14. **Pain onset.** A study by Radnanov found that patients who reported pain immediately after their accidents were more likely to have pain at two years post-injury.[168] It is generally recognized that patients with immediate symptoms are at a higher risk of long-term pain from whiplash.

A careful history is the first step to helping a whiplash patient recover quickly and easily. Now that we have a clear picture of what happens in a whiplash injury, let's look at some of the most common symptoms of whiplash.

Chapter Two
Symptoms

Neck Pain

Whiplash injuries are basically simple. During a collision, the head and torso are thrust in opposite directions in a very short period of time. So it is not surprising that most of the symptoms of whiplash are centered in that part of the body between the head and the torso—the neck.

Radanov[119] cites a 97% rate of neck pain after whiplash injury in chronic patients. Greenfield et al[162] and Deans et al[26] report that the onset of neck pain occurs in 65% of patients within six hours, within 24 hours in an additional 28%, and within 72 hours in the remaining 7%.[37]

Etiology

The cervical spine contains many important structures, and as we saw in the section on biomechanics, is susceptible to trauma. The following is a description of the different anatomical structures that have been shown to suffer injury from whiplash-type impacts.

Myofascial Trauma

Myofascial damage is by far the most common source of neck pain in whiplash injuries. Evans[37] wrote: "The vast majority of whiplash injuries result in cervical sprains, i.e., myofascial injuries." Friedmann et al[45] state, "Muscular strain in the cervical area can be extremely complex. The large number of small muscles in the region have different functions in different head positions. It is an area quite subject to strain. It may be difficult to distinguish between sprain, strain, and nerve root involvement."

Luo and Goldsmith[90] found that the splenius capitis muscle can be stretched more than 30% in a whiplash injury, giving some idea of the amount of myofascial damage that can be done.

Pearce[309] reported on a case of a woman who suffered severe swallowing pain after she suffered a fall. The author attributed the symptoms to damage of the longus cervicis colli.

Croft[21] writes, "As the head rotates into hyperextension, the anterior cervical muscles are stretched, and when their tone is overcome, the brunt of the remaining force is taken up by the anterior longitudinal ligament and anterior fibers of the annulus fibrosus. If the rate of stretch of these muscles is rapid, individual muscle fibers may not have sufficient time to relax. This results in rupture of muscle."

Croft[21] also sheds some important light on the flexion portion of the injury, and the damage that can occur in the suboccipital region of the spine: "...the upper cervical spine sustains the greatest injury, as it tends to be the biomechanical pivot point. I would agree with these findings and submit that it is because of this and the fact that the muscles in this region, i.e., suboccipital and occipitofrontalis muscles, are smaller and more specialized that they are

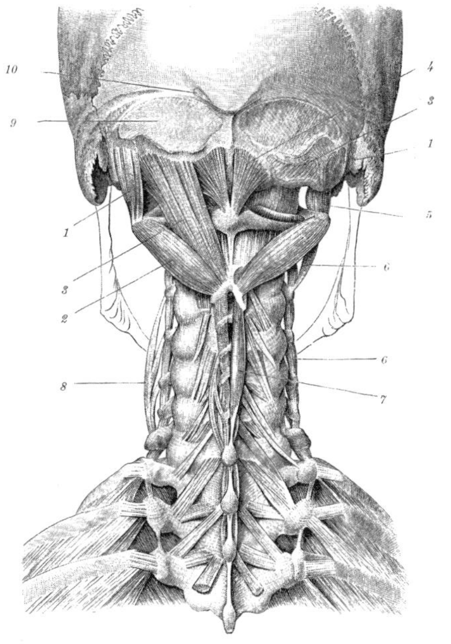

Figure 10.
The small muscles of the upper spine may be susceptible to injury during the flexion phase of whiplash.

so commonly traumatized to a greater degree than the larger paraspinal muscles." [21] (See Figure 10.)

In 1964, MacNab[91] performed a landmark study in which he used primates to analyze the exact trauma experienced during whiplash injuries. On examination post-injury, he found damage to the longus colli and sternocleidomastoid muscles. These findings were confirmed with MRI by Davis et al.[24] Also susceptible to trauma are the scalenes, especially during the extension phase.

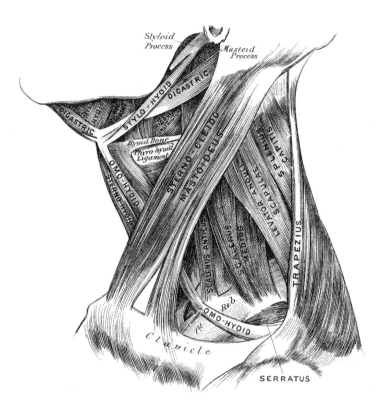

Figure 11.
The neck is made up of dozens of muscles. The anterior strap muscles, including the sternocleidomastoid and the scalenes, are the most susceptible to injury from stretching during the whiplash motion.

Studies by Szabo et al[385] and McConnell[289,290] have consistently reported anterior neck pain in whiplash test subjects, further documenting the role these muscles play in whiplash pain (Figure 11).

Myofascial trauma in the cervical spine can be responsible for many other symptoms of whiplash besides neck pain. In 1938, Kellgren[73] found that injections of a salt solution created specific patterns of referred pain for different muscles. Referred pain from soft-tissue damage in the neck can cause pain in seemingly unrelated parts of the body. For instance, trigger points in the levator scapulae muscle can cause referred pain down the back and into the shoulder, as well as cause symptoms down the arm and into the fourth and fifth fingers.[145,158] Headache can also easily be a result of referred pain, especially with trigger points in the upper trapezius (Figure 12 and 13).[31]

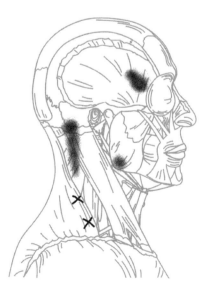
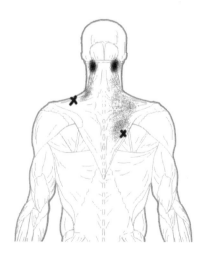

Figure 12 and 13.
Trigger points of the trapezius marked with X, referred pain in shaded areas.

Fredin et al[218] suggested that the excess muscular tension they found in whiplash patients originated from the joints of the cervical spine, rather than the muscle tissue itself.

> "Mechanical stimulation of joint capsules of the knee and ankles and increased tension in cruciate ligaments have been found to change the activity of the muscle spindle afferents, indicating that ligaments and probably capsules play an important sensory role. The receptors in the ligaments and capsules may contribute to the regulation of muscular stiffness around the knee via reflex actions on the gamma muscle spindle system and thereby to the control of joint stiffness and joint stability. It is likely that receptors in capsules and ligaments play a part in the regulation of muscular stiffness and tension also in the neck."

Ligamentous Damage

Dorman[28] wrote, "Would it be simplistic to suggest...that the cause of pain in whiplash injuries after rear-end collisions is from injury to the ligaments and fasciae in the neck?"

Since most of the forces that cause a whiplash injury are those experienced during the extension phase, it is not surprising that the ligaments of the anterior portion of the spine are susceptible to trauma. The most commonly recognized ligamentous damage is tears of the anterior longitudinal ligament (Figure 14). Dvorak et al[33] also found evidence with CT scans of damage to the alar ligament. Most of the damage to the ligamentous structures seems to be focused between C4 and C7,[37,92,281] where most of the forces

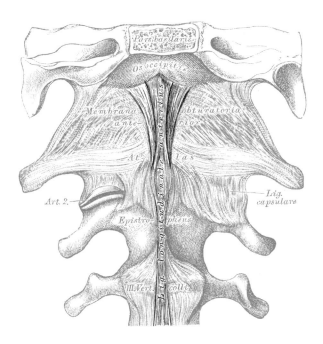

Figure 14.
The anterior longitudinal ligament, shown highligted, is a thin band of tissue that runs along the front of the spine. This ligament may be damaged when the spine hyperextends.

are centered during hyperextension.

Davis et al,[24] in a comprehensive evaluation of patients with MRI (Magnetic Resonance Imagery) scans also found damage to the anterior longitudinal ligament, as well as trauma to the posterior interspinous ligament. Gebhard et al[50] state that, "complete disruption of ligamentous support," is rare. Actual ligament tearing would most likely occur during higher speed collisions (>10 m.p.h.).

Further evidence of ligamentous damage after whiplash is provided by Otte et al.[305] They found abnormalities in the brains of whiplash patients, but concluded that the changes in brain structure were not due to direct head trauma. "[I]t may be that the perfusion deficits are caused by ... a mechanism in the upper cervical spine."

Disc-Related Trauma

Connective tissue damage of the spinal column is well documented in the medical literature as a result of rear-end accidents. Davis et al[24] found horizontal avulsion of the vertebral end plates, separation of the disk from the vertebral end plate, acute posterolateral cervical disk herniations, and prevertebral fluid collections. Figure 15 shows a cross-section of the cervical spine, with details of what types of trauma have been found on diagnostic exams.

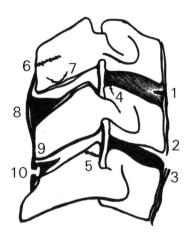

Figure 15.
Spinal Injuries
1. Rim Lesions
2. Endplate avulsions
3. Tears of the anterior longitudinal ligament
4. Uncinate process
5. Articular process
6. Articular pillar
7. Articular subcondral fractures
8. Haemarthrosis
9. Haemmorrhage into a meniscoid
10. Capsule tear of the zygapophysial joint

While studies have documented the existence of connective tissue damage as it relates directly to the spine, diagnosis of these lesions can be difficult.

Bogduk[11] wrote, "Most of the lesions underlying the pain of whiplash are occult and are not detectable using conventional techniques. Standard CT scans, myelography and EMG are of no value unless neurological signs are evident...They show only spinal compression or nerve root compression, which are rare in whiplash and which should already be evident on clinical examination."

The issue of isolating the exact lesion in the cervical spine is not made easier with MRI, according to a study by Pettersson et al.[115] In this study, 39 whiplash patients were examined an average of eleven days after their accident. "26 of these showed changes on MRI with disc lesions in 25, 10 of which were classified as disc herniations..." Thus 26 of 39 patients (67%) had findings on MRI; previous studies done on asymptomatic patients have found that only 19% of pain-free necks have spinal abnormalities. "Thus it seems that patients sustaining whiplash injuries of the cervical spine have a higher than normal frequency of MRI findings." Interestingly, although 26 of the 35 patients had neurological signs, these signs did not correlate well with the location of the lesion on MRI findings. The researchers in this study concluded that lesions of the cervical spine are more complex than simple neurological "impingement" of the nerve roots.[115]

Facet Joint Injury

Over the last few years, researchers have focused a great deal of attention on the role of facet joint injury caused by whiplash accidents.

Figure 16 and 17.
Areas of pain caused by injury to the facet joints.[220]

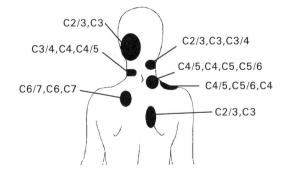
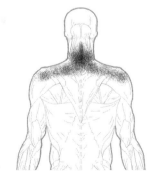

Fukui[220] described the pain patterns associated with zygapophysial joint pain (Figure 16). As you can see, this pattern of pain is nearly identical to the pattern of pain described by Squires[341] (Figure 17).

Lord et al[269] studied this issue further, and injected the nerves that innervate the facet joints with either anesthesia or saline (Figure 18). They found that the patients who were injected with the anesthesia showed a much greater relief of pain than did the placebo subjects. They concluded that 50-60% of whiplash patients showed strong evidence of facet joint injury.

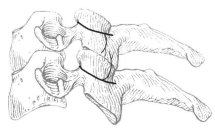

Figure 18. Nerves that innervate the cervical facet joints.

A later study by same group of researchers[271] studied the effect of radiofrequency neurotomy on the same nerves. Neurotomy entails "cooking" the nerves that lead from the facet joints with an electrode at a temperature of 176° F (80° C). The study found that 7 of 12 patients reported relief from pain symptoms. This led the authors to conclude again that the facet joints play an important role in whiplash pain. Unfortunately, the treatment was only about 40% successful in the long-term, and patients needed repeat treatments to maintain their pain-free status.

They wrote, "Although we have shown that percutaneous radio-frequency neurotomy is significantly more efficacious than placebo, problems with the procedure remain. Despite apparently clear diagnoses, patients may obtain no relief even after more than one neurotomy. Others can have additional pain revealed after their original, dominant pain is treated."[271]

Yet another study by Wallis et al[360] reported in another study using radiofrequency neurotomy that when the physical pain was relieved from the technique, the psychological symptoms vanished immediately.

Degenerative Changes

Whiplash injuries can lead to degeneration of the spine. Evans[37] states, "There is evidence suggesting that trauma and whiplash injuries can accelerate the development of cervical spondylosis with degenerative disk disease." This is substantiated by a number of studies. Hamer et al[58] reported that "whiplash injury causes cervical changes predisposing to premature degenerative disc disease." This is echoed by Kenna and Murtagh:[75] "In the long term the disc rupture will lead to degeneration of the intervertebral disc with narrowing of the intervertebral space and osteophyte formation." Hohl[67] found degenerative changes in 39% of a group of whiplash patients, five years after the injury.

Petterson et al[311] performed MRI on 39 whiplash patients within 11 days of whiplash injury, and compared these findings to the MRIs in the same patients two years later. The study found that a total of 13 patients (33%) had disc herniations that were graded as moderate or severe. "The majority of disc herniations were at C4-C6, which is in accordance with findings in previous studies, indicating that this is the most stressed segment."

"Persistent symptoms developed in five of six patients with grade 3 disc herniation, and three patients were still on sick-leave at the follow-up examination 2 years after trauma compared with 1/14 of patients with no disc pathology. This demonstrates a possible association between the whiplash injury and cervical disc disease as was recently proposed."[311]

Boden[181] added that these patients with disc abnormalities (at the two-year follow-up) were 2.7 times more likely to have symptoms than those patients without lesions.

Neurological Trauma

We can break down neurological symptoms of whiplash into two different categories: indirect nerve involvement and direct lesions of nerve tissue.

Indirect Nerve Damage

The function of the nervous system in the human spine can be affected by any of the above-mentioned traumas. Probably the most familiar in this category is that caused by disc herniation, which can put pressure on the nerve roots, leading to radiculitis, shoulder symptoms, headache, or arm pain, depending on which nerve root is involved. Disc herniation is an indirect source of irritation or damage to the nerve, as these nerves are not injured from the collision directly, but from herniations caused by the accident.

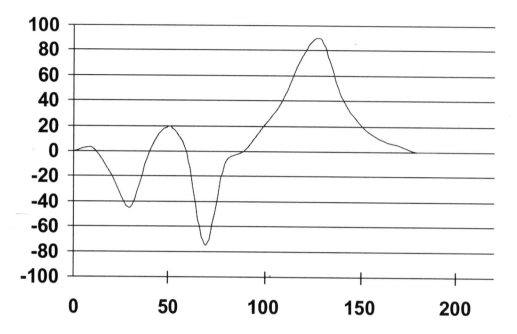

Figure 19. Spinal pressure changes dramatically during whiplash motion.

Another method of indirect nerve damage has been suggested. Ortengren et al[301] studied the effects of whiplash motion on pigs, and found a dramatic increase in cerebrospinal fluid pressure during such motion (Figure 19). The authors write,

> "Aldman[171] predicted that transient pressure changes would occur in the central nervous system during swift extension-flexion motion of the human cervical spine. The spinal canal alters its length and thus its inner volume during this type of movement. This induces alterations of the blood volume of the epidural vein plexa. Venous blood is forced to flow along the spinal canal and through the bridging veins in the intervertebral foramina. When the neck motion becomes rapid, as for instance during whiplash extension motion, so will the flow of vein blood. Pressure gradients will arise due to flow resistance and due to the acceleration of fluid mass. Such pressure gradients are expected to rise over the intervertebral foramina and are likely to add to the load caused by mechanical movements of the tissue inside the foramina. Injuries to the spinal ganglia may thus be a consequence. Such a mechanism for the induction of injury would explain several of the symptoms that are known to be claimed by patients exposed to neck extension trauma (whiplash)..."

Of interest is the fact that one of these first pressure pulses occurs at exactly the same time as the newly discovered S-shape curve appears during the whiplash motion. Other researchers have studied the effects of trauma on ganglion nerves.[344,371] This is a new area of study on whiplash, and may provide further insight into whiplash-injury mechanisms in the coming years.

Direct Nerve Damage

Concussion is one example of direct damage to the nervous system (see Brain Injury).

The cervical sympathetic nerve trunk lies directly anterior to the longus colli, and like that muscle, may be susceptible to trauma during the extension phase of whiplash. Stretching of these nerves is believed by some to result in Horner's Syndrome, nausea, dizziness, blurred vision, and tinnitus.[37,45,75]

The occipital nerve can be directly crushed between the bony arches of the atlas and axis during sudden hyperextension.[81,182,273] (For more information, see Occipital Neuralgia under headache.)

Bodack et al[180] reported on a single case of spinal accessory nerve palsy (SANP) after a whiplash accident. The authors state that patients with SANP commonly complain of arm heaviness and moderate pain in the shoulders, possibly shooting out to the neck and arm. The intensity of the pain is usually heightened if the shoulder is unsupported, or if the patient is carrying or lifting heavy objects. Also, if the shoulder is elevated above its resting height during daily activities, pain may be experienced. To compensate, patients rely heavily on forward flexion of the torso and elbow flexion to accomplish the normal use of the shoulder. "A sudden acceleration-deceleration event involving the cervical spine, as occurs in a typical whiplash injury, may subject the SAN to a very large force of stretch over a very rapid rate of time. The SAN is more prone to injury if the head is turned to the contralateral side prior to the event, as the ipsilateral nerve is put on stretch in this position."

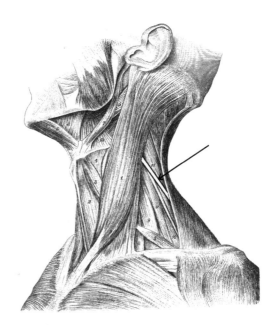

Figure 20.
The spinal accessory nerve can be stretched during a whiplash injury.

Skeletal Trauma

Serious fractures of the cervical spine during whiplash are rare.[11] It is well-documented, however, that small fractures of the vertrabrae can occur in severe whiplash injuries. These include fractures of the articular pillar, articular process, and the uncinate process (Figure 15). Barnsley et al[7] have documented damage to the zygapophysial facet joints from whiplash injuries. All of these fractures can be difficult to identify and may be responsible for long-term pain.

Vascular Damage

The exact frequency of vascular damage after whiplash is not known, but there are studies that show that it does occur. Friedman et al[44] found that 24% of patients with severe cervical trauma (not limited to whiplash, but including whiplash) were found to have abnormal vertebral artery findings.

MacNab[91] stated that "...spasm of the vertebral arteries might explain in some instances the etiology of tinnitus, deafness, and nystagmus."

Giacobetti et al[226] performed magnetic resonance angiography on 61 patients admitted to a hospital with cervical spine trauma. The authors found that "complete disruption of blood flow through the vertebral artery was demonstrated...in 12 of the 61 patients (19.7%)." Flexion injuries were found to be the most common type of injury in patients with vertebral artery injury.

Nibu et al[297] performed an experiment with cadaver spines, and reported that the vertebral artery could experience elongation during even low speed impacts.

Viktrup[354] reported a case of stroke that occurred in a patient who showed signs of vertebral artery damage after whiplash.

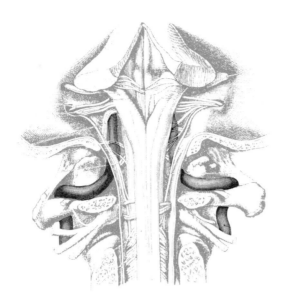

Figure 21.
The vertebral artery, shown highlighted, may be injured during rapid motions of the upper spine.

Injury to the vertebral artery is probably due to the fact that it follows a circuitous path through the upper cervical vertebrae. Severe, rapid motions in this segment of the spine could easily stretch the artery excessively (Figure 21).

Imaging Cervical Trauma

One of the most difficult things about whiplash injuries is that traditional radiography rarely show traumatic lesions.[384] Techniques such as CT scans and MRI offer new tools in the search for pathological changes after whiplash.

Van Goetham et al[352] provide the following summary on the efficacy of radiographs, CT, and MRI in the diagnosis of whiplash injuries::

- Plain radiographs: "Plain radiography is the first imaging technique that should be used in patients who sustained a whiplash injury. This is not only to evaluate possible traumatic lesions, but also to have a reference image of the cervical spine at the time of the trauma. This way secondary lesions, such as degenerative disease, can be objectively assessed when they are recognized some time after the trauma." The authors also warn that, "Plain radiographs have a low sensitivity for identifying traumatic cervical spine lesions. In a large series of patients[368] with cervical injuries, the combination of cross-table lateral (CTL), AP and OM-views missed 61% of all fractures, 36% of subluxations and dislocations and falsely identified 23% of the patients, half of whom had unstable cervical injuries, as having normal cervical spines. Therefore, trauma victims with plain films positive for cervical injury, or negative for cervical injury but with a high clinical suspicion of injury, should undergo CT or MRI for a more definitive evaluation of the cervical spine." [352]
- CT scans: "CT is indicated in all acute trauma patients when there is no optimal visualization of the cervical spine on plain film, when unexplained focal neck pain or a neurologic deficit exists with a negative plain film, when there is unexplained pre-vertebral soft tissue swelling or whenever the plain film is abnormal…CT is also able to show soft-tissue abnormalities such as disk herniation, soft tissue hematoma and sometimes ligamentous rupture. CT however has definite limitations in evaluating cervical trauma. Increases in intervertebral distances, abnormal angulations, subluxations and dislocations are less well visualized in comparison with plain radiography or tomography. In one study[369] CT only detected 54% of dislocations and subluxations in trauma victims." [352]
- MRI: "MRI findings in whiplash injuries are very diverse and are different depending on the time interval between imaging and the accident.

  "In the chronic phase, more than 1 year after the original trauma, findings are mostly non-specific and include degenerative disk disease, disk protrusion and herniations. Only a minority of patients show bony or ligamentous lesions.

  "In the subacute phase, within 4 months of the whiplash trauma, more characteristic findings such as separations of the disk from the vertebral end plate and ligamentous lesions are reported. The anterior longitudinal ligament (ALL) is more often injured than the posterior longitudinal ligament (PLL) or interspinous ligament…

  "In the acute phase, within 15 days after the original trauma, no specific findings are made."

  "Indications for MRI after whiplash injury include myelopathy, radiculopathy, progressive neurologic deficit, spinal cord injury and an unexpected level of signs above the level of radiographically seen injury…MRI should probably also be used in all patients with whiplash injury who have persistent complaints or significant findings at any other investigation, since these patients have a worse prognosis and may exhibit significant MRI findings."[352]

Benzel et al[178] reported that MRI was much more reliable than CT scans. While 62 patients showed evidence of soft-tissue injury on MRI, CT scans only detected two patients with abnormalities. They state, "The posttraumatic cervical syndrome (whiplash) is a widespread and costly problem about which little is understood. The information presented here indicates that the MR imaging findings of paraspinous soft-tissue injury may suggest such an entity. In fact, they may be an imaging correlate of the whiplash syndrome for which the establishment of a clinical/imaging correlation has not been achieved previously. Perhaps a review of early post-injury MR images may provide insight into the etiology, and potentially the management, of persistent posttraumatic neck pain."[178]

MRI abnormalities in the cervical spine, however, are not proof that the lesions were caused by the whiplash accident. Wood et al[367] performed MRIs on 90 symptom-free subjects and found that 73% of them showed evidence of abnormalities, including herniations, bulging discs, and annular tears. The authors state that MRI-detected soft-tissue lesions are only meaningful if accompanied by corresponding objective signs.

C-Reactive Protein

Pritchett[315] discussed the use of a C-reactive protein test to detect occult soft-tissue injury. The study found that patients with tendon or ligament tears had CRP levels of 4.1 (mg/dL) for acute disc rupture, 9.2 for anterior cruciate ligament tear, and 10.1 for Achilles tendon tear, 48 hours after the injury. Patients with pain but no tearing had CRP levels below 1.0 mg/dL. The levels of CRP in tear groups remained above 1.1 mg/dL even after two weeks.

The author explained the significance of these findings: "C-reactive protein is synthesized by hepatocytes in response to interleukin-6 secreted by macrophages at the site of tissue injury…C-reactive protein levels have been determined to be <1.0 mg/dL in 99% of normal healthy subjects. Following a variety of procedures and injuries such as joint replacement, tibial fracture, major trauma, disc excision and spinal fusion, the serum CRP level can increase several-hundred-fold."

A test of serum CRP may be a useful tool for detecting occult ligamentous or tendon tissue damage that does not appear on radiological tests after cervical or lumbar spinal trauma. The CRP test in this study cost $22, making it affordable. Physicians interested in using this test should note that CRP levels lag behind the traumatic event, and the test may not be effective until 48 hours after the trauma.[315]

Treatment

Conservative treatment of neck pain is widely recognized as the best approach. Conservative medical treatment of neck pain consists of bed rest, analgesics, NSAIDs, muscle relaxants, or sleeping medication. Narcotic analgesics are occasionally prescribed for neck pain.[37,88]

Some practitioners still prescribe a cervical collar.[145] Mealy et al[163] found that early mobilization of the neck was more effective at treating whiplash pain than was rest or a cervical collar.

Teasell and McCain[145] have this to say about cervical traction: "Traction has been advocated by some authors, but in our experience cervical traction often aggravates symptoms in both the acute and later stages…Traction is not a substitute for a proper stretching program."

Direct soft-tissue manipulation can be very effective at treating the myofascial component of neck injuries. Teasell and McCain[145] state, "Massage therapy is a time-honored treatment for musculoskeletal problems, in particular myofascial pain and increased muscle tension."

Injection of botulinum toxin has been attempted in such patients with cervical myofascial pain syndrome. Hobson and Gladish[242] reported that an injection of botulinum toxin into the localized tender area of the left trapezius muscle resulted in a reduction from 1 headache a week to 1 to 2 headaches per month, and the severity of the attacks was considerably reduced. The headaches returned within 3 to 4½ months after the treatment, necessitating injections of botulinum toxin every three months for the last three years.

Chiropractic

A recent RAND study by Hurwitz et al[245] found that chiropractic treatment shows effectiveness in treating acute neck pain as result of whiplash, and that it was also safe.

Beneliyahu[8] reported on the benefits of chiropractic manipulation in the treatment cervical disk herniation.

In a more recent study that used MRI to follow the course of chiropractic treatment of herniated discs, Beneliyahu[176] reported, "...that 22 of 27 (80%) had good clinical outcomes; 17 of the 22 (77%) "had not only good clinical outcome but also evidence of reduced or resolved disc herniation upon repeat MRI scanning."

In a small study done by Woodward et al,[370] the researchers found that 93% of whiplash patients improved with chiropractic care—even when the outcome parameters were measured by an orthopedic surgeon.

Rogers[325] also recently studied the use of chiropractic in the treatment of whiplash. He found that his spinal manipulation patients showed a 44% improvement in pain symptoms on average, while a group of stretching patients showed just a 9% improvement. In regard to proprioceptive functioning, similar results were found: a 41% improvement in the manipulation group, but only an 11% improvement in the stretching group. How spinal manipulation affects proprioception is not yet known, but Rogers speculated that chiropractic treatment somehow stimulates the deep articular mechanoreceptors in the spine, in turn leading to improved functioning.

Koes et al[78,79] also reported that for nonspecific neck and back pain, spinal manipulation was more effective than care by a general practitioner.

Surgery

Surgery for whiplash neck pain is sometimes performed on patients with chronic pain, but has not been found to be very effective.[58] Algers et al[1] found that of 20 patients who were operated on for chronic whiplash symptoms, only 2 had good results, 9 had fair results, and 9 had poor results. The authors state, "Thus, in spite of extensive diagnostic evaluation, it is difficult to identify the painful segment in patients with persisting symptoms after whiplash injury. The diagnostic difficulties might be one explanation of the unsatisfying operative results in our series as well as in others." Algers et al[1] make it clear that these findings do not represent malingering on the patients' part, but that the disc protrusions seen on radiological tests may not be responsible for the pain.

Conservative treatment is considered the standard, even in cases with documented herniation of the cervical disc. Saal et al[331] studied a group of 26 patients with herniations who were treated conservatively. One year later, 92% of the patients were still working full-time, with 88% in the same job. "Twenty of 24 nonoperative patients had a good or excellent outcome," or 83%. "No patients had progressive neurologic loss or reached a neurologic catastrophe (i.e., new onset of myelopathy)." Two patients had surgery. The authors concluded, "Until there is a randomized clinical trial comparing surgery and nonsurgical care, it is important to consider that aggressive nonoperative care is indicated in every cervical disc herniation patient before a decision for surgical intervention."[331]

Sometimes herniations heal spontaneously. Westmark et al[362] reported on a case of a woman who had a number of serious cervical spine herniations documented by MRI and was scheduled for surgery. She changed her mind on the day of surgery, however, and was not seen for two years. At that time, she was given another MRI and the authors found that three of the herniations had resolved significantly, without treatment..

MultiModal Care

The latest literature shows that a multidisciplinary approach is often the best way to treat whiplash. Provinciali et al[316] studied two groups of whiplash patients—one received a multi-modal approach that included relaxation training, psychological support, and direct soft-tissue treatment (massage and mobilization); the other group received TENS and ultrasound treatment only. They found that the multimodal treatment patients recovered faster, reported less pain, and returned to work earlier than the TENS and ultrasound patients did.

Headache

Post-traumatic headache is a major problem in our society. Ham et al[57] state that "Each year it is estimated that 1.4 million people in the United States are head-injured; of these individuals, approximately 30-50% will develop chronic headaches which persist for more than six months."

Headache is the second most common symptom of whiplash, only after neck pain. In the acute stage, Wiley[154] has found a incidence of 97%. In chronic cases, Radanov[119] found a prevalance of 78%, and Balla et al[6] reported a rate of 82% in their studies of whiplash patients.

A large number of studies show that organic pain may be at the root of whiplash-related distress. Wallis et al[179] state that there is substantial evidence that whiplash headache is real and that physicians need "...to resist the temptation to ascribe whiplash-associated headache to situational stress and 'tension,' and, instead, to consider the possibility of an organic pain source."

The symptoms of headache are obvious. Not so obvious is the fact that a variety of different headaches can arise from whiplash injury. The following is a summary of these different types of headache.

Cervicogenic Headache

A growing body of literature has examined the role of the cervical spine in the origin of headache. Sjaastad et al[378] provide the following diagnostic criteria for cervicogenic headache:

(I)   Symptoms and signs of neck involvement:
    (a) Precipitation of head pain, similar to the usually occurring one:
        (1) By neck involvement and/or sustained awkward head positioning, and/or:
        (2) By external pressure over the upper cervical or occipital region on the symptomatic side
    (b) Restriction of the range of motion (ROM) in the neck.
    (c) Ipsilateral neck, shoulder, or arm pain of a rather vague nonradicular nature or, occasionally, arm pain of a radicular nature.
(II) Confirmatory evidence by diagnostic anesthetic blockades.
(III) Unilaterality of the head pain, without side-shift.

For clinical diagnosis, patients must exhibit at least one of the phenomena in section I. The more criteria the patient fits, the more appropriate the diagnosis.[378]

Occipital Neuralgia

Most headaches from whiplash are considered to be "cervicogenic" or arising from the cervical spine. Occipital neuralgia is a specific type of cervicogenic headache that involves damage or pressure on the occipital nerve. "Greater occipital neuralgia can be caused by a direct blow to the suboccipital region or by an entrapment by the semispinalis capitis." [37]

Magnusson et al,[277] in a study of 15 patients with intractable whiplash headache wrote that, "The GON [greater occipital nerve] has been shown to penetrate the trapezius muscle in many individuals raising the possibility of irritation or trauma to the nerve as it pierces the muscle. In whiplash trauma,

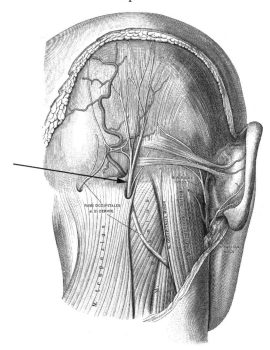

Figure 22.
The occipital nerve can be entrapped by the trapezius, resulting in headache pain.

forcible bending of the neck occurs, possibly combined with neck traction when the head is thrown forward or sideways by accelerating/decelerating forces. This kind of trauma can, therefore, put a strain on the GON, especially in the case of anatomic entrapment. In most individuals, the GON pierces the semispinalis muscle of the head and compression of the nerve at that level seems possible."

Another source of potential nerve damage is the crushing of the C2 spinal roots (Figure 23). LaBan[81] states, "Unlike other spinal nerves, the ganglia of the C2 spinal roots lie exposed on the vertebral arch of the axis. In this position they are vulnerable to crushing between the bony arches of the atlas and axis during forced hyperextension of the head. Additional complaints include severe headache in the retro-orbital, temporal, and parietal, as well as occipital, areas, scalp 'cramps,' and burning dysthesias, which may be described by patients as 'my hair is on fire.' "

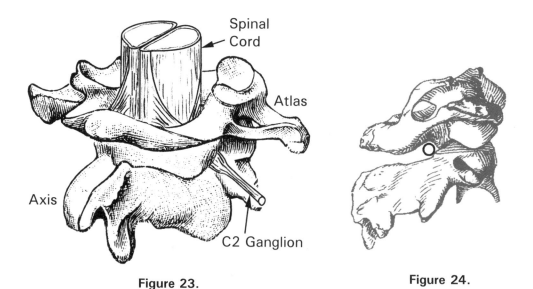

Figure 23.   **Figure 24.**

Lu and Ebraheim[273] performed an anatomical study that lends credence to the notion of cervicogenic headache—specifically, headache arising from entrapment of the C2 nerve root ganglion. Fifteen cadaveric spines were examined, and the authors measured the height of the foramen (the space between the C1 and C2) and the height of the ganglion.

The authors found that the C2 ganglion occupies, on average, 76% of the space provided by the foramen. Figure 23 shows the atlas, axis, and C2 nerve root ganglion (Figure 24).

From their anatomical findings, the researchers suggest that the C2 ganglion is particularly susceptible to compression, resulting in damage to the nerve and headache.

"Considering these results, the authors believe that the anatomic features of C2 ganglion may predispose to its vulnerability to compression. In the report of his cadaveric study, Bogduk[182] noted that during rotation combined with extension (i.e., whiplash injury), the posterior arch of the atlas and the superior articular process of the axis were approximated sufficiently to contact the C2 ganglion. The C2 ganglion, the thickest neural structure, is the most susceptible to compression."

The authors further state that, "It is likely, therefore, that the cervicogenic headache occurs as a result of displacement, abnormal movements, or arthritic changes in the atlantoaxial joint where the C2 ganglion and nerve root are compromised."

Poletti[313] studied six patients with third cervical root ganglion compression after whiplash accidents. C3 compression was diagnosed by location of symptoms (i.e., "from the neck, up behind and over the ear…"); headaches described as "sharp," "shooting," "jolts," and "jabs;" numbness in the C3 dermatome; and worsening of symptoms upon cervical motion.

The exact frequency of occipital neuralgia is not known, and the issue is complicated by other factors. Graff-Radford et al,[54] however, warn that "occipital neuralgia and myofascial pain may produce a similar clinical picture, [and] it is emphatically recommended that examination for myofascial trigger points be carried out in all patients with clinical pictures of occipital neuralgia."

The problem of confusing occipital neuralgia with myofascial referred pain has been reported by others. Radanov et al[123] found that "Trauma related headache was described as arising in the occiput projecting to frontotemporal." They also found that "The quality of pain did not fulfill criteria of any defined neuralgia." Thus, a careful examination is necessary to determine appropriate treatment of the headache.

Myofascial Headache

Most headache pain is attributed to myofascial trauma. Evans[37] stated, "Headaches following whiplash injuries are usually of the muscle contraction type…" Duckro[31] wrote that, "…myofascial irritation is a significant contributing factor in chronic post-traumatic headache." The important point to keep in mind with these types of headache, however, is that the pain may originate in a variety of different places in the head, neck, and back.

Referred pain *from damaged myofascia is the most common source of tension headache,* particulary in the occipital region of the head. The occipital region contains many delicate structures, and muscle swelling or spasm as a result of whiplash can affect the occipital nerve, leading to pain. Muscular or ligamentous damage in this area of the spine can also cause referred pain to other parts of the head.[31,54,145] For more detailed information, please consult Travell and Simons.[158] (See Neck Pain.)

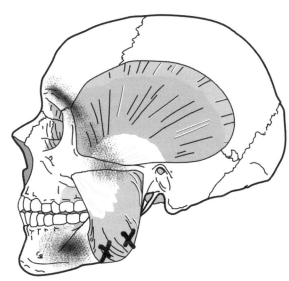

Temporomandibular Joint Dysfunction *(TMJ or TMD)* is another possible source of headache pain.[146] TMJ pain is documented thoroughly in the literature as a sequela of whiplash-type injuries, but is often overlooked as a source of headache. Muscular tension in the jaw can cause referred pain to other parts of the head[158] (Figure 25). (See Temporomandibular Joint Dysfunction.)

Figure 25. Trigger points in the jaw, marked with an X, can cause headaches in the shaded areas.

Blunt trauma directly to the soft-tissue of the neck or head can also lead to myofascial damage, and subsequent headache. It is important to investigate whether the patient hit his or her head at the time of the collision. It may be that simple myofascial damage occurred and is responsible for the head pain, but it is also important to rule out the possibility of mild traumatic brain injury. (See Mild Traumatic Brain Injury.)

Stress is a familiar source of muscular tension. With the all of the different stressful events that a whiplash patient must endure, it is not surprising that tension headaches could arise after such an accident.

Migraine

Teasell and McCain[145] state that, "In our experience common migraine headaches are not uncommon following whiplash injuries and often occur in individuals with no previous history of migraines."

Migraine headaches are a poorly understood condition. Some researchers speculate that they may arise from a vascular dysfunction; others suggest a neurological causation.[146] With this much controversy over common migraine, it isn't surprising that there are even more disagreements about post-traumatic migraine. In fact, many physicians don't consider post-traumatic migraine to be a real condition. Pearce, a long-time opponent to the idea of whiplash itself[113] states in an editorial, "Migrainous features are not the result of whiplash injury." [114]

A thorough reading of the literature, however, leads to a much different conclusion. Evans[37] states, "Whiplash injuries can occasionally precipitate recurring common, classic, and basilar migraines de novo. The headaches can begin immediately or within a few days after the injury."

Jacome[69] reported the occurence of basilar artery migraines after whiplash.

Weiss et al[153] evaluated 35 patients with post-traumatic migraine, seven of whom had been in a whiplash accident. None of these patients had a history of headache, or signs of brain lesions. "The headaches began within hours to days of the injury." The study found that, contrary to the theory of compensation neurosis, the headaches did improve with treatment, and compensation did not extend the period of disability. All of the patients in this study previously had been given "muscle relaxants," with no improvement. The authors used migraine medications for treatment (propranolol and amitriptyline) but, "After several months of successful treatment, headaches recurred in 10 patients when the amitriptyline or propranolol was withdrawn." [153]

This recurrence of headaches suggests that the underlying pathology was not treated. Other researchers have provided some insights into why traditional migraine therapy does not completely alleviate the symptoms. Teasell and McCain[145] state the situation clearly:

> "Traditionally, tension and migraine headaches have been regarded as entirely separate entities, with differing characteristics, mechanisms, and treatment. However, the distinction may not be so apparent in clinical practice since there may be overlapping features between tension and migraine headaches. The clinical spectrum of benign, recurrent headache appears to include classic migraine at one end, the variations of common migraine and tension-vascular headache occupying the middle ground, and tension headache at the other end."

Raskin[159] suggests that the entire spectrum of whiplash induced headaches—including migraines—has a cervicogenic basis. The myofascial origins of migraine-type headaches have recently been substantiated by three recent studies. Blau et al[9] in an analysis of fifty patients with migraine, found that 32 subjects reported neck pain directly related to the migraine symptoms. They wrote, "This study shows that neck pain or stiffness is a manifestation of extracranial involvement during all phases of migraine episodes." Kidd and Nelson[77] also reported that myofascial dysfunction of the neck seemed to play a role in migraine and tension headaches. Duckro et al[30] found that migraine headaches can be related, or even result from, low back pain. The authors state that migraine headaches may result from "dysfunctional patterns of muscle use" and that the "development of painful muscles...at the upper back and neck may contribute to the development or exacerbation of migraine headache."

Mild Traumatic Brain Injury

Mild traumatic brain injury is a complex and controversial issue that is dealt with in greater depth in Chapter Four.

Gilkey et al[227] wrote, "Headache is the most common neurologic symptom following minor closed head injury. There is often a lack of objective evidence supporting an organic basis of cerebral pathology in these cases."

Gilkey and associates compared 35 post-traumatic headache sufferers with 92 patients with migraine and 49 non-headache control subjects. The cerebral blood flow of all participants was measured, using the "xenon Xe 133 inhalation technique." This imaging method involves the detection of a radioactive gas (Xe 133) inhaled by the subject, which shows the flow of blood through the brain.

The researchers found significant differences in blood flow between the post-traumatic headache patients and the migraine and nonheadache control subjects. The authors explain how this abnormal blood flow is related to brain injury:

> "Traumatic brain injury does not mechanically tear axons but rather causes focal intra-axonal change that leads to progressive axonal swelling and ultimately leads to disconnection. These pathobiological changes impact on the normal functioning of a cell, as well as neurotransmitters, neuromodulators, and electrical brain activity. This can result in interference with the regulatory capacity of the central, peripheral, autonomic, and vasomotor systems, impacting on CBF [cerebral blood flow]." [227]

Diagnosing headache that results from mild traumatic brain injury can be very difficult. Landy[262] reported on two cases of post-traumatic headache that are of interest:

The first case was a 40-year-old man who had been hit in the face during a fistfight, and sustained a concussion. He had no other neurological signs, and a CT scan was normal. One month later, however, the patient "returned with increasing headache, nausea, and lethargy. A new CT scan showed bilateral subdural hematoma."

The second case was of a 42-year-old woman who fell on the right side of her head. A CT scan was done in the emergency room, and was normal. One month later, with signs of cortical dysfunction and complaints of headache, an MRI was performed. It found a "small subacute hemorrhage in the left temporal lobe consistent with a contrecoup injury."

Other Headaches

There are primarily three other types of headaches that have been identified as related to whiplash injury. They are: vascular, sympathetic, and drug induced.

Vascular Headaches. Packard and Ham[111] state that after mild head injury, "Cerebral circulation is often abnormal," and that, "In many patients, the cerebral circulation is slowed for months or even years after injury, and this may accompany prolonged post-traumatic symptoms." As mentioned in *Neck Pain: Vascular Damage*, the vertebral artery can be damaged in whiplash injuries, potentially creating headache symptoms, although the exact frequency of headaches from such trauma is not known. Nibu et al[297] reported that the vertebral arteries of cadavers showed excessive stretching during whiplash motion. Vijayan[160] has proposed that traumatic stretching of the carotid arteries may also cause headache.

Sympathetic Nerve Dysfunction is another potential source of headache pain. Khurana and Nirankari[76] reported on two cases of posttraumatic headache where the suspected cause was damage to the cervical sympathetic nerve trunks. (For a more in-depth treatment of nerve damage, please see the section Neck Pain: Neurological Damage.)

Analgesic Rebound Headaches are another important issue. Many patients with whiplash injury are taking medications for pain. Ironically, overuse of analgesics for pain are a well-documented source of headache, and some drugs cause headaches as a side-effect.[88] These headaches are known as *analgesic rebound headaches*. Rapoport et al[319] found that 73% of patients with rebound headache were women, and was most common in patients aged 31 to 40 years. "Eighty percent of respondents indicated that depression was commonly observed in analgesic rebound headache sufferers; 77% indicated that physical conditions (especially gastrointestinal symptoms) were commonly observed." All patients should be evaluated for this possibility of analgesic rebound headache. (For more information on adverse drug reactions, see the Medications section.)

Prognosis and Treatment

Parker and Rosenblum[307] have identified the following areas that should be evaluated in these posttraumatic headache patients: "consciousness, sensorimotor, neurophysiological, cerebral personality disorders, general intelligence, memory, language, information processing, post-traumatic stress, indentity, adaptation, and developmental problems of children."

Conservative treatment should be adequate for most whiplash-induced headaches. Chronic headaches, however, if left untreated are unlikely to go away on their own, as some patients still have symptoms many years after the injury.[122,123]

Traditional treatment of headache pain consists mainly of drug therapy.[146] Once serious pathological lesions have been ruled out, there is little the medical profession can do for chronic headache patients.

Graff-Radford et al[54] made an interesting statement about invasive treatment of headache believed to be neurological in basis: "To date, the most common treatments for occipital neuralgia have been neurally destructive surgical procedures...however, patients often report feeling worse after such procedures."

Magnusson et al[277] wrote that surgical release of the occipital nerve may be indicated, but only in a highly selected group of patients.

Poletti[313] found in his patients with 3rd cervical root ganglion compression that at least half of the patients required further surgical intervention for recurring symptoms, and the author concluded that, "As with other compressive radiculopathies, all efforts should be made to treat patients conservatively."

Some types of headaches may require medications for proper management. For tension headaches, however, Gobel et al[51] found that amitriptyline may reduce pain, but it does not resolve the underlying muscular tension.

As mentioned earlier, the myofascial approach to headache is gaining more acceptance. Cyriax[23] wrote, "The fact that pain in certain parts of the head might originate from distant points had long been apparent to me clinically as a result of the search for the spots massage of which relieved the patient's headache." Cyriax believed strongly in the direct application of massage to the trauma: "Massage must be given daily until the symptoms have gone...Provided the correct spots are massaged firmly and persistently there should be next to no failures." He also stressed the importance of direct work on the cervical muscles.[23]

Of course, massage is not the only treatment for posttraumatic headaches. For example, Boline et al[12] recently reported that spinal manipulation demonstrated better long-term management of tension headaches than did amitriptyline. Any modality that directly heals affected tissues should be very successful at relieving headache pain that originates in the connective tissue.

Fibromyalgia

Fibromyalgia affects an estimated 1 to 5% of the population.[116,193] Ledingham et al[83] and others have reported that 15% of fibromyalgia patients attribute the onset of their condition to trauma.

Diagnostic Criteria

The American College of Rheumatology (ACR) developed a diagnostic protocol for fibromyalgia in 1990. The ACR diagnosis is:

1. A history of widespread pain for more than three months, and
2. Pain in 11 of 18 tender points upon palpation (see chart and Figure 26).[155]

Location of Tender Points
- Occiput
- Low Cervical
- Trapezius
- Supraspinatus
- Second Rib
- Lateral Epicondyle
- Gluteal
- Greater Trochanter
- Knee (Not shown)

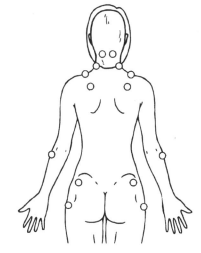

Figure 26. Tender points used to diagnose fibromyalgia.

The diagnostic criteria are general, and may include many different chronic pain conditions. Croft et al[22] addressed this problem, stating, "The combination of chronic widespread pain and high counts seemed to be one end of a spectrum of pain status and tender point counts rather than a distinct entity."

Etiology

Fibromyalgia is a well-recognized symptom of whiplash injury, but is also surrounded by controversy. Teasell and McCain[145] wrote: "A particularly frustrating group of patients are those with a typical whiplash injury who, rather than gradually improving, actually seem to progressively develop a generalized chronic pain state identical to the fibromyalgia syndrome. Patients with whiplash injuries often meet established criteria for fibromyalgia."

Fibromyalgia seems to be a condition closely related to injury of the neck. Buskila et al[193] studied two groups of injury groups: one group who had suffered neck injury and another who had suffered leg injuries. There were no differences in litigation between the two groups. Fibromyalgia, however, was **13 times** more common in the neck injury patients than in the leg injury group.

The problem with fibromyalgia is that researchers have been unable to identify a specific pathology responsible for the condition. For years, researchers looked only at the affected muscles, assuming that the pain was originating in those tissues that were painful. Research has moved away from specific muscular pathology, and has increasingly examined the role of the nervous system.

The most recent research on fibromyalgia has focused on disturbances in the central nervous system (CNS). McDermid et al[291] reported generalized hypervigilance in FM patients, and Wachter et al[357] recently published a study that found evidence of hyperactivity of the sympathetic nervous system in patients with fibromyalgia and other pain syndromes.

Further evidence that fibromyalgia may be a systemic problem has been put forth by two groups of researchers.

Rosenhall et al[326] reported that fibromyalgia patients exhibit symptoms indicating dysfunction of either the brainstem or the cervical spine itself. They suggest that the dysfunction found in fibromyalgia patients may actually be a result of disturbed neck proprioception. Proprioceptive damage has also been linked to whiplash injuries.

Griep et al[234] found in their 1998 study that fibromyalgia patients had significant disturbance of the hypothalamic-pituitary-adrenal axis, or the stress response system. Similar dysregulation has been found in patients with PTSD, depression, and chronic fatigue syndrome.

In a similar vein, Amir et al[172] found that in a group of 29 PTSD patients, 20% also fit the diagnosis for fibromyalgia. The authors write, "...Kuch et al[80] found that, among 60 patients treated for fibromyalgia syndrome in a pain clinic, the prevalence of phobias and PTSD were 3.2 times more common in victims of minor road vehicle accidents than in subjects with non-vehicular-related onset of pain...The present study indicates that fibromyalgia syndrome has a substantial overlap with PTSD, which supports the psychological background of the disorder."

What this latest research seems to indicate is that fibromyalgia, and perhaps whiplash itself, is a phenomenon that is not related just to the neck, but the entire nervous system.

Fibromyalgia or Malingering?

Chronic myofascial pain is considered by some to be malingering. The medical research dispels this myth. Waylonis and Perkins[151] investigated patients with post-traumatic fibromyalgia, to see if there were any differences between them and patients with idiopathic fibromyalgia. They found that fibromyalgia symptoms continued long after litigation had been settled, and that there were no statistically significant clinical differences between post-traumatic fibromyalgia and idiopathic fibromyalgia patients.

Romano[124] studied the effect of litigation on post-traumatic fibromyalgia as well, and worked from the assumption that if fibromyalgia patients were malingering, they "probably would not continue to see their treating physicians after a monetary award was granted...(i.e. they would 'take the money and run')." In this series of 14 patients, ten (71%) continued to see a rheumatologist on their own after the settlement was reached.

Moldofsky et al,[101] in another study, also reported that finalizing litigation did not reduce pain levels. A 1996 study by Turk et al[351] compared a group of posttraumatic fibromyalgia patients to patients with idiopathic fibromyalgia. The traumatic onset fibromyalgia patients reported more pain, distress, disability, and lower general activity than the idiopathic-onset fibromyalgia patients did. However, the authors report that, "The greater disability and psychological distress in the post-traumatic [fibromyalgia] patients were present even when we controlled for compensation status, a potential mediator. Thus, the differences between the two types of [fibromyalgia] onset cannot be attributed solely to a desire by these patients to receive some financial gain."

Fibromyalgia and Misdiagnosis

There has been some concern that patients are diagnosed with fibromyalgia when in fact they have another condition with similar symptoms.

Smythe was one of the original physicians involved with creating the diagnostic guidelines for fibromyalgia in 1990. In a 1994 study[136] he details the clinical features and treatment of a related phenomena—one that can be confused with fibromyalgia.

The C6-7 Syndrome results from tenderness in the area between the cervical vertebrae C6 and C7. "While the intertransverse spaces are often tender, the maximum tenderness affected the bone and attached structures at the anterolateral corners of the vertebral bodies; exactly where radiological examination will show osteophytes late in life. The localized tenderness long precedes radiographic change." [136]

Again, as we saw in the Biomechanics and in the Neck Pain section, this region of the spine takes the brunt of trauma during low speed collisions.

Soft-tissue tenderness was also present in the "medial epicondyle, at the origin and insertion of pectoralis minor (i.e. the 4th or 5th rib inside the anterior axillary line), and at the tip and medial aspect of the coracoid process." The tenderness in these regions resulted in diffuse referred pain in the upper body that could easily be mistaken for fibromyalgia.

In this study, the patients were instructed on how to use a cervical pillow to relieve the strain on the affected tissues. After eighteen months using the cervical pillow, 63% of the patients (all of whom had bee originally diagnosed with fibromyalgia) were improved.

Tenderness and trigger points in the pectoralis minor after whiplash were also found in a study by Hong and Simons.[68] Specific treatment of the pectoralis minor resulted in relief of symptoms (Figure 27).

A study by Fitzcharles and Esdaile[216] found a high rate of fibromyalgia diagnosis in a group of women with unrecognized spondyloarthopathy.

Chronic whiplash itself may provide a diagnosis of fibromyalgia, since the tenderpoints used to diagnose fibromyalgia are virtually identical to the patterns of pain exhibited by whiplash patients.

These studies show the importance of a careful examination before a diagnosis of fibromyalgia is given.

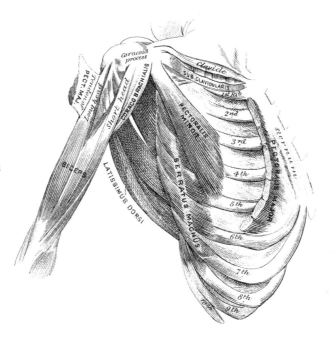

Figure 27.
The pectoralis minor may be responsible for symptoms similar to fibromyalgia.

Treatment

Treatment of fibromyalgia is difficult.[116] Some studies have found that regular exercise is useful as a treatment, but many patients with fibromyalgia find it difficult to exercise because of the pain. Getting the patient started on simple, enjoyable exercise (such as walking or swimming) can be very helpful. Strenuous exercise has not been shown to be beneficial, and may be more frustrating for the patient because of physical limitations.

Medications have been extensively used for fibromyalgia, but for most patients the benefits have been modest and offset by adverse drug reactions.[116] Many of the drugs that are commonly used for fibromyalgia are sedatives, such as: amitriptyline, Valium, Xanax, and Halcion. One study[156] examined the use of fluoxetine (Prozac) in the treatment of fibromyalgia, and found that it was not effective.

Waylonis and Perkins[151] found that post-traumatic fibromyalgia sufferers used a variety of different treatments for their pain. The most common were chiropractic, massage, osteopathy, physical therapy, and biofeedback.

The latest literature shows that a multidisciplinary approach is the best way to treat fibromyalgia.

Mason et al[283] found that an educational/behavioral program was effective at reducing fibromyalgia pain during the course of the treatment, but that improvements were not maintained after the program was completed.

Nicassio et al,[298] on the other hand, found that an educational approach did not help during the course of treatment, but had helped at a six-month follow-up. Pain levels showed no improvement, but the patients did report improved functioning and reduced depression and pain behavior. The key seems to be creating patterns of coping and functioning that the patient can continue over time.

There has been much written in the last few years about the concern of a "disability mentality" that is starting to form in relation to fibromyalgia. One study[365] found that as many as 25% of fibromyalgia patients in the US have received some sort of disability payment or compensation.

Aaron et al[377] found that fibromyalgia patients were much more likely to receive disability compensation if they had a traumatic onset of their condition.

This mentality is most harmful to the patient himself. As Wolfe[366] recently wrote:

> "That FM will always be with us because patients suffer with its symptoms is true regardless of what we name the syndrome. It is possible to improve the lot of those with FM, but first we must take control of our own beliefs about FM as a disease, about the effectiveness of treatment, and about the role of psychological factors. We must halt the trend to label patients with FM as disabled, and we must interfere with the societal trend toward encouragement of the disability concept." [366]

Temporomandibular Joint Pain

Tempomandibular joint (TMJ) disorders after whiplash are well-documented in the literature.[317, 188, 260, 327, 209] Frankel[42] found that 15 of 40 (37.5%) whiplash patients had symptoms of TMJ trauma. More recently, Heise et al[61] reported that in an analysis of 155 whiplash patients, between 12.7-15% of the patients had TMJ symptoms.

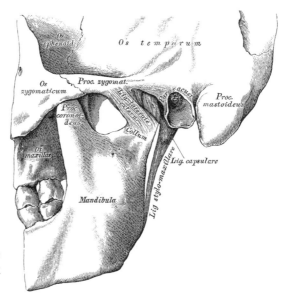

Figure 28. The TMJ is a common area of pain after whiplash injury.

The TMJ is where the mandible connects to the temporal bone of the skull (Figure 28), and involves the joint as well as the numerous muscles that connect both structures.

Lader[82] wrote, "Due to lack of recognition by the patient's health care provider, a traumatic injury to the neck can cause seemingly unrelated symptoms of TMJ dysfunction and chronic headache. Many whiplash injury victims needlessly suffer with chronic intractable pain and eventually manifest permanent degenerative changes in their TMJs."

Garcia and Arrington[222] write, "We can no longer overlook the jaw — MR imaging clearly demonstrates the relationship between post MVA [motor vehicle accident] cervical whiplash and TMJ injuries. Based on the forgoing, an examination of the TMJs for possible injuries should be an integral part of any comprehensive evaluation of post MVA cervical whiplash patients."

The extent of this problem is emphasized by Kolbinson et al:[257]

> "We find it troubling that TMJ symptoms were identified by the patients themselves (rather than by health care providers) for over 80% of the study patients. Nondental health care workers must heighten their awareness of the possibility of TMD-related problems occurring in the MVA patient…"

Signs and Symptoms

Here are the most common symptoms of TMJ trauma:[86,146, 203, 256]

- Joint noises (i.e. popping, clicking, and crepitus)
- Limited range of jaw motion
- Pain in the TMJ region
- Muscular spasm in the jaw
- Referred pain to other areas of the head (Figure 29)
- Headache
- Retro orbital, bitemporal, and occipital pain
- Shoulder pain
- Tinnitus

Etiology

Levandoski[86] breaks down the etiology of TMJ pain into two categories: macrotrauma and microtrauma.

"Macrotrauma usually occurs from a single acute event that disturbs the TMJs." Macrotrauma from whiplash can be direct, such as hitting the jaw on the steering wheel, or indirect, which can "occur when the victim is in a motor vehicle accident,

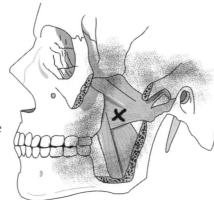

Figure 29. Trigger points deep in the jaw can create pain throughout the head.

wearing seat belts, and the upper body is tossed about with sudden extreme high velocity, multi-directional, wrenching, and overextension injuries to the TMJs and upper body." Macrotrauma is the most common source of TMJ pain: "Anywhere from 80 to 95% of a TMJ disorder patient population will eventually recollect some form of significant macrotrauma..."

"Microtrauma," Levandoski[86] writes, "is a low grade chronic or repetitive type of injury that constantly subjects a part of the body to over-loading abuse." Sources of microtrauma from whiplash can include "the prescription of cervical collars, unprotected cervical traction, extraction trauma, [and] fixation immobilization to reduce fractures."

Although whiplash-induced TMJ dysfunction is well-recognized in the medical literature,[152] the exact mechanism of trauma in non-contact injuries in not known. Some researchers have postulated the existence of "mandibular whiplash"—or a dramatic opening of the jaw during a collision that could cause damage to the TMJ. More recent studies[199] have discredited this theory, and experimental collisions involving human test subjects[290] have failed to show any evidence of excessive jaw motion during collisions at speeds of 7 mph. Roydhouse,[126] however, provides an interesting observation: "Car seat belts usually have a diagonal shoulder-restraining component. This restricts movement of the upper torso but for convenience it usually has an extension system that locks only if the extension is above a certain speed, as in a sudden forward movement...The rapid imposition of restraint by the diagonal belt in a vehicle occupant who is thrown forward can lead to a burn on the side of the neck or to bruising...The presence after an accident of a bruise or burn on the left side of the driver's neck or jaw...may be related to general head pain. This pain appears to asymmetric; the body of the jaw is painful on one side, while the temporomandibular joint and temporal muscle are painful on the other. In one case the victim had chipped teeth; the belt restraint had forced the mandible upwards and sideways."

Any force that can chip teeth without direct head contact could seemingly result in damage to the TMJ.

Research by Goldberg et al,[231] using SPECT imaging, suggests that TMJ patients may have something in common with mild traumatic brain injury patients. Although the size of their study group precluded statistical analysis, "there were some intriguing trends that suggested underlying central nervous system changes in a subset of patients."

> "...although patients with a documented loss of consciousness were excluded from this investigation, it is conceivable that they may be similar to patients with concussion-related disorders, given the marked preponderance of the aforementioned symptoms [i.e., irritability, anxiety, depression, poor memory, poor concentration] as well as the test results reported in this study. Although it cannot be concluded unequivocally that [posttraumatic TMJ] population has indeed suffered a mild brain injury, or concussion for that matter, the potential similarities between this population and the mild traumatic brain injury population should be studied further."

Burgess et al[192] found that higher speed collisions were more likely to result in TMJ problems than were lower speed collisions. However, they also found patients were more likely to have TMJ pain if they had their head turned in either direction at the time of the collision, or if their car was hit from the rear. Turned head position is a risk factor for increased risk of injury during a collision. The study also noted that a large percentage of the TMJ patients were women—89%. Delayed onset was also a problem addressed: 15% of the patients reported that the symptoms appeared one month or longer after their accident.

Contradicting this study is a more recent study by the same group of researchers that found that patients involved in minimal vehicle damage accidents reported more treatment visits and had higher rates of tenderness than with severe damage.[257]

After assessing the accident and impact factors, the researchers found a slower recovery in those collisions with: minimal vehicle damage, lack of headrest use, poor driver position, and settlement of claim. This last finding is particularly interesting, as litigation is usually believe to prolong symptoms: "…insurance claim settlement at the time of the initial visit did not seem to suggest a better prognosis for patients with post-MVA TMDs…"[257]

Another study by Kolbinson et al[255] interviewed 30 posttraumatic TMJ patients and found that 73% of the patients had their insurance claim or litigation settled for an average of 21 months. However, 23 patients (76.7%) reported that they still had symptoms from their injury, and 8 (26.7%) felt that their jaw symptoms interfered with their daily activities. Only 8 reported that they had no more jaw pain, but two of these reported some pain since the settlement or in the last 3 months. Twenty-three patients (76.7%) reported that they had headaches, and 25 (83.3%) stated that they currently had neck pain.

When the patients were divided into those with current litigation and those who had settled, the researchers found virtually no difference between the two groups in terms of symptoms—in fact, the group of patients with settled claims reported slightly more neck pain than those with pending litigation.

It is quite possible that TMJ pain after whiplash is not due to any unique mechanism during the collision, but is a result of a more general tension that occurs as a result of trauma.

Treatment

There is a strong concensus that conservative treatment for TMJ is the best approach. If the TMJ pain is of soft-tissue origin, as most of it is, traditional medical treatment consists of a "soft, chewy diet; the application of heat to the joint; Valium as a muscle relaxant and tranquilizer; analgesics." Splints are often prescribed by dentists. Psychological stress is recognized by many physicians as a possible source of TMJ pain, and counseling is usually recommended.

The soft-tissue of the jaw and the TMJ itself cannot really be separated from one another — they are clearly part of one functioning unit.[203] Even in cases where articular damage is present, there is usually muscular spasm. Therefore, the use of soft-tissue therapy should be considered in the treatment of TMJ pain, especially before considering surgery. If the pain is articular in origin, more invasive procedures are used, including surgery.[146]

In one surgical study, Steigerwald et al[342] found that many TMJ surgical patients reported an immediate relief of pain following surgery, even though most of the patients had been in pain for about six months. Especially interesting was the finding that after surgery, "…not only did the muscles relax and become nontender, but trigger points were inactivated as well, possibly explaining some of the cases of immediate resolution of headache and dizziness." In short, many of the myofascial symptoms disappeared after surgery. Unfortunately, surgery only reduced pain levels, and did not eliminate the pain entirely.

MultiDisciplinary

The latest literature reports that a multi-disciplinary approach is much more effective in treating TMJ pain than the tradional medical approach. Kolbinson[256] reported that 40% of the trauma patients had the same number of symptoms at the end of treatment as they had at the beginning. In a study by Greco,[233] only 3.5% had no change in symptoms. Greco used a combination of splint therapy, biofeedback, and stress management. Even more impressive was the fact that treatment in the Greco study was limited to a series of six sessions, but was ongoing in the Kolbinson study.

Manipulation

Martini et al[282] reported on their use of manipulation in the successful treatment of TMJ pain. "In 1500 treated cases, documented on videotape, only five cases required surgical intervention. The success of the therapy was confirmed by 13 MRI images of the TMJ of patients with acute and chronic locking before and after therapy. In all cases the anteriorly dislocated disk in closing and opening position was recaptured and repositioned in a normal position in the tempormandibular fossa."

The Martini's manipulative reduction technique is described as such: "The patient is instructed to relax and slightly open the mouth as much as possible before pain occurs. The clinician is positioned behind the patient. The patient's head is turned away from the locking side (in cases with bilateral locking, to the most recent locked side). The clinician places his thumb right on the lower dental arch of the locking side, left or right. The other hand is placed on the temporale of the same side in order to stabilize the patient's head during the manipulative maneuver. The distal phalange of the thumb is flexed and the joint of the second phalange contacts the upper arch at the molar level, functioning as a fulcrum. The power of the lever is expressed by the third, fourth and fifth finger positioned on the lower border of the mandibular body."

"Light pressure is applied on the lower second molar. The pressure is applied in a back and down direction and is increased inward as the condyle is freed of interference with the disk. The hand stabilizing the head applies a progressive pressure in the opposite direction to the hand on the teeth and inclines the head forward. At the same time, the clinician moves the mandible in an antero-medial direction."

"The index finger of the stabilizing hand, pushes the condyle out of the fossa and compresses the empty fossa when the mandible is opened. The manipulative reduction maneuver must be painless (with no clicking)."

The authors also detail physiotherapeutic exercises that the patient does after the manipulation to assist in healing the TMJ. "This mandibular manipulation is dependent upon the clinician's technical ability. It requires adequate training (1-2 months) before a health care provider becomes sufficiently clinically skilled."

Thoracic Outlet Syndrome

Capistrant, in a review of 64 consecutive whiplash cases, found symptoms of thoracic outlet syndrome in 33%.[15] Sanders and Pearce[128] examined a series of 491 thoracic outlet syndrome (TOS) patients and found that 56% of the cases were caused by automobile accidents. Moore,[293] in 1986, found that 33% of whiplash injury patients reported arm symptoms which he related to TOS.

The symptoms of TOS include: aching pain in the shoulder or arm; heaviness or easy fatiguability of the arm; tingling and numbness in the ulnar aspect of the hand, especially the 4th and 5th fingers; finger stiffness; edema of the arm or hand; coolness and pallor of the hand. Neck tightness and headaches in the posterior region of the head are also common.[117,127,138,146]

Diagnosis

The following tests are used to diagnose TOS.

- **A positive Tinel's sign.** For this test, pressure is applied to the brachial plexus for 10 to 60 seconds. If positive, the patient's symptoms may appear, including numbness in the hand.
- **The Roos test** is another useful test for TOS. In this test, the patient hyperabducts and externally rotates the arms, while opening and closing his or her hands (Figure 30). If positive, the patient's symptoms will appear.

For more definitive testing of TOS, there are a variety of electrodiagnostic tests that check for impaired nerve conduction or compression of the blood vessels.[127, 138]

Etiology

Roos and Owens[125] wrote, "Any injury causing a severe 'jerk' of the shoulder or neck may precipitate the outlet syndrome, including the so-called 'whiplash' auto injury. Arm symptoms may not develop for several days, weeks, or even months after the injury; however, they tend to be relentless and poorly responsive to physical therapy when they do develop."

Mailis et al[278] found that 67% of the TOS symptoms in a group whiplash patients were on the side of the driver's shoulder strap, suggesting that the force of the body against the shoulder restraint during whiplash may be responsible for TOS symptoms.

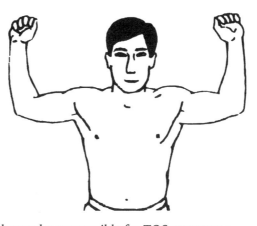

Figure 30.
The Roos test for diagnosing TOS.

A variety of different forces can affect the nerves and blood vessels of the thoracic outlet. Arterial or venous compression are both rare (less than 2% of all cases.) Neurogenic TOS is equally uncommon. 90% of all cases of TOS are classified as "symptomatic."[127] These cases have no objective findings, and are therefore subject to accusations of malingering. Evans[37] states that nonspecific TOS "can also be considered as an anterior cervical strain resulting from a whiplash injury to the scalene muscles, which causes referred paresthesias from trigger points rather than from neurogenic irritation."

The myofascial component to TOS is echoed in other studies as well. Ellison and Wood[35] wrote, "Scalene muscle injury secondary to trauma is emerging as the most common aetiology of thoracic outlet syndrome. The theory is that a patient sustains an injury, most commonly a hyperextension injury to the neck in a motor vehicle crash, which results in haemorrhage and oedema in the region of the scalene anterior and medius muscles. Following injury, fibrosis and contracture of the scalene muscles occur."

Sanders[127] discusses the existence of increased fibrosis in the scalenes of TOS patients, and states, "Any entity that causes swelling and/or fibrosis of the scalene muscles can elicit symptoms of TOS." He goes into more detail about how whiplash injuries can cause the symptoms of TOS: "Anatomical dissections in the operating room and labora-

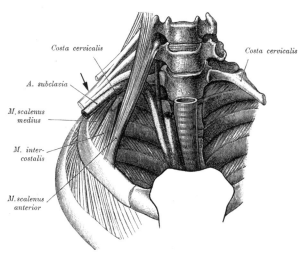

Costa cervicalis

A. subclavia

M. scalenus medius

M. inter-costalis

M. scalenus anterior

Costa cervicalis

Figure 31.
The thoracic outlet. The brachial plexus (shown by the arrow) is at risk of being trapped between the scalene muscles.

tory have revealed that the nerves of the brachial plexus usually pass through the narrowest part of the scalene triangle, where there is no space...Following trauma, if these muscles have been tightened or hardened by an inflammatory process, it is easy to envision how these nerves could be irritated and produce neurologic symptoms."

The brachial plexus is susceptible to entrapment, as it passes through the "scalene triangle," as seen in Figure 31).

Prognosis and Treatment

As stated earlier, Roos and Owens[125] reported that TOS symptoms can easily become chronic.

Medical treatment usually consists of muscle relaxants, analgesics, and physical therapy. Surgery is often used in chronic cases, and it usually consists of removal of the first rib.[127] Surgery is not a guaranteed solution, as Ellison and Wood[35] found that only 27% of patients were completely recovered after surgery; 52% had almost complete pain relief, but with continuing impairment; and 21% still had considerable disability. Lindgren and Oksala[87] followed 45 TOS surgery patients for 21 years, and found that only 43% of the operations were successful. These authors state, "It may be asked how big the placebo effect of surgery is and whether it has been taken into account, considering that the success rate of surgery is low." They also state that in regard to adverse effects of TOS surgery, "neurologic deficits, brachial plexopathies, causalgias, and even deaths have been reported."

A more recent study by Lindgren,[268] reported, "the results after surgery are no better than a placebo effect, a fact that is overlooked...According to the present study, conservative therapy is the treatment of choice in TOS because it is safe and can be implemented as a self-treatment program."

Sucher[138,139] described a much more conservative approach to the treatment of TOS. The first component is patient self-stretching of the scalenes, illustrated in Figure 32. In this stretch, the patient sits, with the arm on the side to be stretched secured down by hooking it under the seat. The patient then takes the other hand and wraps it around the head, pulling it over as much as tolerated, leaning the body away from the stretched side. He also advocates stretching of the pectoralis minor. This stretching is designed to loosen those tissues that are impinging on the structures that move through the thoracic outlet.

The second component of Sucher's technique is direct myofascial release work of the scalenes and pectoralis minor.[138,139]

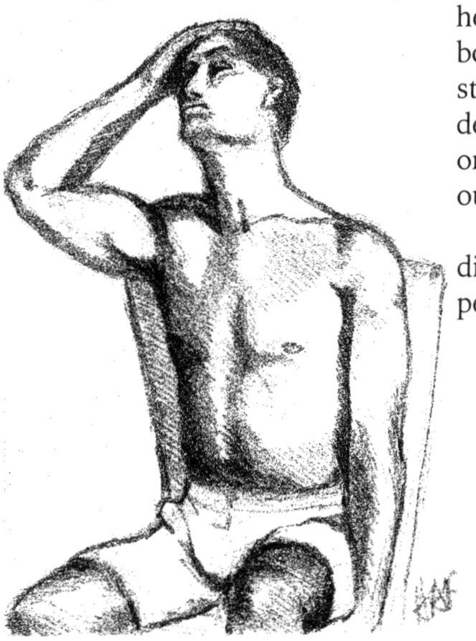

Figure 32.
Stretching of the neck musculature can help release pressure on the thoracic outlet.

Low Back Pain

Low back pain after whiplash injuries is common. Radanov[119] reports the prevalance of back pain after whiplash as 42%. Wiley et al[154] found a rate of 60%. Hildingsson and Toolenan[64] found a back pain incidence of 25%, two years after the injury.

Etiology

The lumbar spine is more stabilized in whiplash accidents than is the cervical spine. Whereas the head is free to rotate, flex and extend, the lower back is held against the seat. Most of the damage to the low back in whiplash is due to the fact that the pelvis is held immobile by the seat belt, and the torso is allowed some degree of movement. In automobiles with only lap belts and without shoulder restraints, this movement of the spine is even more pronounced. A soft seatback can also allow the lumbar spine to experience more severe hyperextension than a firm seatback.[37]

Wiley et al[154] suggested that the cause of pain in the low back after whiplash was a sprain of the lumbar ligaments. Teasell and McCain,[145] however, state, "The pain is typically myofascial, with multiple trigger points noted along the ischial crests, quadratus lumborum and paravertebral muscles, upper sacroiliac joints, and sacrum." (See Figures 33-35.)

The myofascial origins of low back pain after whiplash was supported in a study by Grable.[53] In this study, ninety patients with low back pain after motor vehicle accidents were given MRI scans. Twenty-four of these patients, or 27%, were found to have abnormal MRIs. Boden[10] examined the MRIs from 67 people with no history of low back pain and found a prevalence of abnormal MRIs of 28%. Jensen et al[71] also reported similar findings. This strongly suggests that the abnormal findings on MRI scans seen by Grable are not significantly more than those in asymptomatic subjects. If neurological signs are present, however, then more serious pathology may be responsible for the symptoms and this should be carefully investigated.

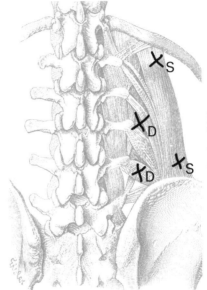

Figure 33.
Trigger points in the quadratus lumborum can refer pain to the hip and buttocks. Deep points shown with D, superficial points shown with S.

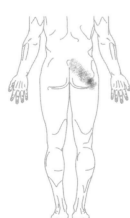

Figure 34.
Area of referred pain from deep trigger points of the quadratus lumborum.

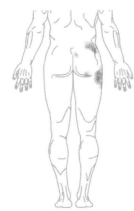

Figure 35.
Area of referred pain from superfical trigger points of the quadratus lumborum.

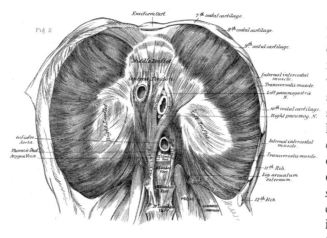

Figure 36.
The diaphragm attaches at the 3rd and 4th lumbar vertebrae, where most lower back degeneration occurs.

Another possible cause of low back pain involves the diaphragm. Cisler,[19] in describing the moment of the accident, wrote, "The accident victim suddenly experiences terror and surprise, accompanied by a huge gasp of air with the diaphragm, the largest muscle of the body, reacting to the event; this reaction is termed *shock*." Any traumatized muscle can remain hypertonic, including the diaphragm. The insertions of the diaphragm are along the 12th rib and the 3rd and 4th lumbar vertebrae (Figure 36). 47% of disc degeneration occurs at L4.[147] Chronic contracture of the diaphragm, with the resulting forces on the spine, should be considered in the treatment of low back pain.

Another potential source of low back pain is from the legs. Some whiplash patients brace their legs against the floor of the car when they see an accident coming. Depending on the force of the impact, these forces may traumatize the soft-tissue of the legs and buttocks, causing pain.

In all of the tests done on low speed collisions with live human subjects, only one study has reported back pain as a symptom.[386] In this study, one person stated that they had minor back symptoms after the test impact, and the authors speculated that this may be due to the compression of the spine that occurs early in the collision. With higher speed collisions, back pain may be caused by even greater compressive forces, or, in some instances, the seat back may break. The actual biomechanics of high speed collisions (>10 mph) have not been studied in live human subjects, however, and the exact mechanism of back pain is not yet known.

Symptoms

The obvious symptom of damage to the lumbar spine is, of course, low back pain. There are other symptoms, however, that are less obvious. Some of these symptoms are very important, because of the possibility of serious pathology of the spine.

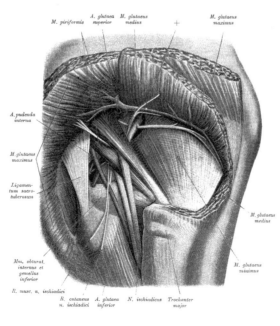

Figure 37.
The sciatic nerve can be impinged by the piriformis muscle, resulting in leg pain.

Sciatica (pain radiating down through the buttocks and along the back of the leg past the knee) can be caused by the piriformis syndrome (Figure 37), or it can be due to a lesion of the intervertebral disks of the lumbar spine.

Fractures of the lumbar spine are rare from whiplash injuries, and they can be ruled out with radiological examinations.

Visceral trauma referring as low back pain is important to consider. Low back pain of this type tends to be constant, worse at night, and not improved by rest. If the patient suffered some kind of abdominal injury in the accident, this could be a serious symptom and should be checked out.[146]

Tingling, numbness, or loss of reflexes of the leg are all indications of disk disease.

Urinary retention or incontinence

is a serious symptom that may mean compression of the cauda equina, and patients with this symptom should be referred to a qualified professional.[146]

Treatment

After reaching a peak a few years ago,[144] low back surgery rates have decreased. Why? Surgery is expensive and has a high failure rate.[34,106] The U.S. Institute of Medicine, in a report on pain and disability, concluded that "surgery for chronic back pain is overused and often misused." [110]

Most low back pain is of soft-tissue origin, but even when the pain is a result of nerve root damage, medical treatment consists of: rest, heat, NSAIDs, muscle relaxants, and oral pain medications.[37,146] If these techniques fail, physical therapy is instituted, and, eventually, surgery. Medications have a general effect, not specifically focused on the origins of the pain.

Direct manipulation of the tissues and the spine are especially beneficial in low back pain treatment. Cisler[19] wrote, "Application of myofascial treatment to the spine, as a whole, assures further that the body benefits throughout from increased improvement of the circulatory system. Such total body treatment may affect and improve the condition of the chronically troubled whiplash patient, as injury sustained in accidents extends beyond the neck region itself. The sooner the initiation of fascial treatment — that is, before chronic changes occur — the better. The body has 'memory of injury,' making injuries tend to become additive."

Melzack et al[96] found that ice massage was just as effective at treating low back pain as was transcutaneous electrical stimulation (TENS).

Chiropractic is recognized as a very effective treatment of low back pain. A RAND study[135] from 1992 cited seven different studies that found that chiropractic manipulation was more effective at treating acute low back pain than was medical treatment. Koes et al[78,79] also found that manipulative therapy and physiotherapy were more effective than medical treatment.

Dysphagia

Dysphagia, or difficulty swallowing, is estimated to occur in about 10% of all whiplash cases.[119]

Etiology

"Dysphagia occurring early after whiplash injury may be the result of esophageal and pharyngeal trauma or a retropharyngeal hematoma. The early occurrence of dysphagia suggests a serious injury likely due to hematoma formation in retropharyngeal structures and is an important prognostic symptom." [145]

In some extreme cases of whiplash, the extension phase of the injury can crush or perforate the esophagus or pharynx.[37]

More likely is soft-tissue swelling or injury adjacent to the esophagus. Pearce[309] wrote about the following case:

"A 42 year old secretary in excellent health fell, in the sitting position, into a stream. She had minor abrasions of the limbs but did not hurt her neck or head. Ten days later she developed a stiff neck. Turning the neck to the left side was painful, making driving difficult. After two days pain increased; prescribed methocarbamol failed to provide relief. On day 3 she had painful difficulty in swallowing, not in the throat but in the right side of the neck 'as if the muscles and ligaments were strained,' and painful movement was relieved when flexing her neck."

The dysphagia increased to the point where the patient could swallow only sips of water. "She held her neck to ease swallowing. She also took to holding her head with both hands to enable her to lay her head on the pillow, and to sit up when getting out of bed." Her symptoms gradually improved, and by day 12 they had resolved.

"The unusual combination of such distinctive symptoms suggests a lesion in the retropharyngeal space involving the prevertebral muscles...The salient features are: (1) The curious location of pain, mainly in the side of the neck. This is quite different from that experienced in common neck sprains of whiplash injury, which are maximal in the posterior neck muscles with radiation to the shoulders, occiput, and interscapular regions. (2) Pain aggravated by movement...(3) Pain is dramatically increased by swallowing. (4) Painful dysphagia is felt not in the throat, but in the side of the neck. Patients may be obliged to hold their necks to allow swallowing. (5) The illness is unaccompanied by fever or systemic disturbance and is self-limiting."

The author attributed the symptoms to damage of the longus cervicis colli.

Treatment

Dysphagia can be a potentially serious symptom if the whiplash trauma was especially severe. If there are doubts, the patient should be referred to a qualified professional.

Carpal Tunnel Syndrome

Carpal tunnel syndrome (CTS) is a fairly common symptom of whiplash trauma.[38]

The most common symptoms of CTS are pain in the hand and wrist. The pain is felt in the thumb, index and middle fingers, and it becomes worse when the wrist is moved. There may also be radiated pain into the arm and shoulder and neck.[72,146]

One very common characteristic of CTS is nocturnal pain. "Up to 95 percent of patients relate a history of awakening in the middle of the night with painful numbness in the hand." [72]

Besides pain, patients also report "electrical" sensations, numbness, and pricking sensations in the hand. Severe cases may exhibit loss of grip strength, swelling, and muscle atrophy.[72,146]

Origins

True CTS is caused by an impingement of the median nerve (Figure 38) in the carpal tunnel of the wrist, but there can be many other problems that can give rise to similar pain.

Neck muscular dysfunction. A fascinating paper by Donaldson et al[381] discusses how disturbances in the tone of the cervical neck musculature can cause CTS. They report that patients with CTS are likely to demonstrate "asymmetric activation" of the sternocleidomastoid muscles on EMG tests. Sternocleidomastoid stretching has been documented in the literature as a result of whiplash biomechanics. They offer an interesting method of treatment that should be examined further (see *Treatment* below).

Cervical radiculopathy. Whiplash injuries can create lesions in the cervical spine.[38] Anatomical studies show that most of the forces in the spine are concentrated on the lower cervical vertebrae.[90] Damage to the nerves at C6 can lead to symptoms similar to CTS.[146]

Thoracic Outlet Syndrome (TOS). Many symptoms of CTS can be actually those of TOS, or the two conditions can exist together, complicating the clinical picture. This condition is referred to as "the double-crush syndrome," because both the thoracic outlet and the carpal tunnel are creating impingement on the nerves. "The term was first coined by Upton and McComas in 1973, who suggested that proximal compression of a nerve might lessen the ability of the nerve to withstand more distal compression."[387] (For more information, see Thoracic Outlet Syndrome.) Swelling of the arm from trauma can also cause symptoms of CTS.[387] It is, therefore, prudent to examine the entire path of the nerve before performing surgery on the carpal canal.

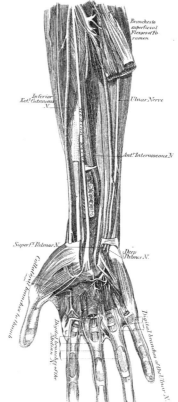

Figure 38.

Trauma of the hand and wrist. Evans[37] stated, "Assuming the symptoms were not preexisting, a hyperextension injury to the wrist while gripping the steering wheel or bracing the hands on the dashboard during the collision could result in carpal tunnel syndrome." Injury to the wrist from airbag deployment is common. If the airbag was activated in the collision, careful examination of the arm is warranted.

Fractures can also be the root of the problem, for instance, if the distal radius or ulna is broken. If direct trauma to the wrist or hand occurred, fractures should be ruled out.[72]

Diagnostic Tests

The following tests can be given for a diagnosis of CTS.

Tinel's sign - performed by tapping the carpal tunnel. A postitive test will cause pain, numbness, and dysesthesias in the areas innervated by the median nerve.[72]

Phalen's test - Have the patient flex the wrist 90 degrees for one minute. A positive test will create numbness and dysesthesias.[72]

Carpal compression test - Press your thumb on the patient's carpal tunnel for 30 seconds. A positive test will elicit symptoms.[72]

Flick test - Ask the patient, "What do you actually do with your hand when the symptoms are at their worst?" In a positive test, the patient will move his or her hand as one would if shaking down a thermometer.[72]

For more accurate diagnosis of CTS, there are a variety of electrodiagnostic tests that will analyze nerve function, but these tests do not necessarily correlate with the patient's symptoms.[72]

Treatment

Conservative treatment is recognized as the best solution for cases of CTS, and it is important that it is started before the condition becomes chronic. Medical treatment consists of NSAIDs, wrist splints, or steroid injections.[146] Surgery is often performed in chronic cases. Surgery carries a risk of complications, however, and Cotton[20] reported that as many as 57% of carpal tunnel release patients experience a recurrence of symptoms two years after surgery. Newer endoscopic surgical techniques are popular, but carry a risk of surgically caused permanent damage.[89]

Donaldson et al[381] offer the following treatment for CTS caused by dysfunction of the sternocleidomastoid (SMC) muscles:

> "The treatment strategy is straightforward in the case of unilateral symptoms. For example, the patient with right CTS symptoms would be treated by focusing on the asymmetrical neck (SCM) muscle imbalance. The treatment protocol, following that described by Donaldson et al[382] would be to have the patient rotate the head to the right and then go into flexion, hold that position for ten seconds, and then return the head to a neutral position and rest quietly for 50 seconds. This would be repeated for a total of six times (i.e., 6 minutes). Three practice sessions in each subsequent 24-h period (for a total of 18 min each day, no more and no less) would be assigned until a restoration of balance is obtained as seen with sEMG..."[381]

Valente and Gibson[149] reported on the benefit of chiropractic manipulation for post-traumatic CTS.

Sucher[139,140,141] has written extensively about the use of specific myofascial release in the successful treatment of CTS. The following is a summary of his technique.

1. " 'Opening' of the carpal canal with stretching and release of the transverse carpal ligament, to increase the space within the canal and thereby decrease the pressure on the median nerve. Pressure is applied centrally from the dorsal surface of the carpal bones simultaneously with pressure applied from the ventral edges of the carpal bones. This is a three-point opposing-pressure system approach. It has the effect of reversing the natural tendency of the 'working' posture to 'flex' the canal and decrease or narrow the carpal space. In effect, the canal is 'extended' and opened up.

   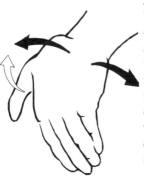

   Additionally, the thumbs pressing on the edges of the wrist bones slide further medially and laterally away from the center of the canal, essentially 'stripping' the myofascial tissue back and enhancing the stretch or release." **Instructions:** Start with the patient's hand as shown in Figure 39. Place your thumbs at the beginning point of the arrows, with your left hand between the index finger and thumb. Your fingertips will press upwards on the bottom part of the hand. Press down with thumbs, up with your fingers in a movement that will open up the carpal canal. With pressure, gradually move your thumbs outward in a stretching movement.

Figure 39.

2. "Release of the true myofascial component of the carpal canal, the attachment of the abductor pollicis brevis muscle. One of the operator's treating hands 'catches' the patient's thumb and pulls it back into hyperextension, with abduction, while simultaneously performing the stretch and release previously described." **Instructions:** Using the same movement as in Step 1, gently hyperextend the thumb.

3. "Indirect stretch of the carpal canal distally, with distension/dilation of the canal internally. The digits and wrist of the patient's involved hand are hyperextended simultaneously with the stretch and release in the first two steps. This hyperextension indirectly stretches the fascia and ligamentous structures over the canal ventrally and especially distally. In addition, the flexor tendons are pulled through the canal so that the more proximal, slightly thicker portion of the tendons (and musculotendinous regions) are actually pulled into the canal and begin to distend the canal from the inside out." **Instructions:** The same movement as in Step 1, but this time hyperextend the patient's hand (Figure 40).

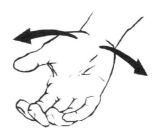

Figure 40.

The patient self-stretch exercise is the same movement, and Sucher has also found this to be effective. The client presses their hand against a wall, as in Figure 41, and presses with the weight of the body. This hyperextends the hand and thumb, and stretches open the carpal canal.

Sucher writes that these techniques can work with chronic cases, but it is easier to get positive results with new cases of CTS.

How do these techniques work? Sucher writes, "…some of the restriction noted on palpation over the carpal tunnel could be due to adhesions or epineural fixations between the median nerve, flexor tendons, and the flexor retinaculum or walls of the canal. It is likely that manipulation and stretching exercises mobilize the nerve by reducing the adhesions."

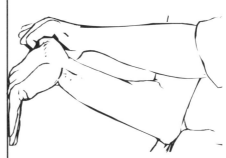

Figure 41.

Gray's Anatomy states that carpal tunnel syndrome, "…is the most common entrapment

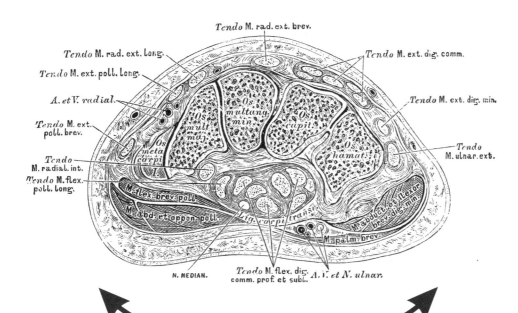

Figure 42.
Cross section of the carpal tunnel.

mononeuropathy and is caused by compression of the median nerve as it passes through the fibro-osseous tunnel beneath the flexor retinaculum. The carpal tunnel may be narrowed by arthritic changes in the wrist joint, particularly rheumatoid arthritis, soft tissue thickening as may occur in myxoedema and acromegaly; and with oedema and obesity including pregnancy. Normally the nerve slides smoothly in and out of the carpal tunnel with flexion and extension of the wrist; when the nerve is compressed there is an additional damage to the nerve with flexion and extesion."

The goal of therapy, as stated by Sucher, is to open and stretch the carpal canal, reducing the pressure on the tissues of the hand, and breaking down adhesions that have developed from overuse or trauma. In Figure 42, you can see what these techniques are attempting to do. The normal state of the wrist is shown here in cross-section. During the stretching maneuver, as shown by the arrows, the carpal canal is 'spread open.' With repeated treatments, the tissues will provide more room for the underlying structures.

Dizziness

Dizziness and vertigo are common symptoms after whiplash injuries. Radanov[119] found a prevalance of 23% in a group of whiplash patients, and Bogduk[11] found a rate of 51%.

Etiology

An excellent review by Fitzgerald[217] discusses the relationship between head trauma and dizziness:

> "For the sake of clarification, the term 'trauma' includes both head blows and whiplash but not injuries severe enough to cause skull fractures or intracranial hemorrhage. No one doubts that head blows, even minor ones, can cause damage to the peripheral vestibular and auditory systems, but many physicians are suspicious of patients with hearing loss and dizziness resulting solely from a whiplash injury. Yet rear-end collisions at only 8 mph generate 5 g of force on the occupant's head. Such force has been shown experimentally to produce injury to the brain stem, cerebral concussion, and cranial nerve stretch in 50% of the monkeys and chimpanzees subjected to it. In reality, many rear-end collisions occur at far higher speeds than 8 mph, greatly increasing the possibility of damage to the CNS and to the peripheral auditory and vestibular symptoms."

There are many possible sources of dizziness and vertigo. The following is a list of the commonly recognized causes.

Mild traumatic brain injury (MTBI), or post-concussion syndrome can be a source of these symptoms, via damage to the inner ear or brain.[37] See the section on MTBI.

Vascular injury, caused by damage to the arteries in the neck and head may also result in "vertebral insufficiency" and dizzness or vertigo.[37] Cases have been reported in the literature of vertebral artery injury after whiplash[226,297] and one case[354] reported stroke after whiplash, resulting in death.

Direct neurological damage. Tamura[143] theorized that nerve root damage in the cervical vertebrae, primarily disc protrusions at the C3-C4 region, may be responsible for dizziness. Similarly, damage to the sympathetic nerves in the neck can also create symptoms. (See Neck Pain section for more details on this type of injury.)

Myofascial damage. There are a number of studies that cite muscular hypertonicity as a cause of dizziness and vertigo. Hinoki[161] found that whiplash patients had abnormal equilibrium tests and suggested that hypertonicity of the cervical muscles may cause confusion in that part of the nervous system responsible for balance. This theory is given support in the work by de Jong et al,[25] who found that when patients were injected with 10 mL of 1% lidocaine in the muscles of the neck, the patients experienced vertigo, difficulty walking, and a feeling of being pulled to the injected side.

Inner ear damage. Mallinson et al[279] reported on a group of patients who showed signs of inner ear damage as a result of whiplash collisions, resulting in vertigo.

Cervical vertigo. This is an area that has seen considerable study since the first edition of this book. This research suggests that damage to the proprioceptive nerves (through stretching of the neck muscles or swelling in the tissues of the cervical spine) can result in dizziness. Proprioception is that part of the nervous system responsible for communicating to the brain the body's movement and position. Proprioceptive receptors in the cervical spine play a key role in the Posture Control System (PCS)—the mechanism by which the body maintains balance and equilibrium. Heikkila and Astrom[240] wrote, "The cause could be functional alterations of the tendinous and the muscular proprioceptors related to the neck muscle function disturbances..." Gimse et al[228,229] reported similar findings, and found that reading difficulties and reduced driving ability after whiplash could be attributed to dysfunction of neck proprioception. Similar findings have been reported by other researchers.[328]

Treatment

Although rare, it is important to rule out the existence of more serious neurological or vascular damage with symptoms of dizziness. If you have concerns about a patient's symptoms, please refer to a qualified professional.

If the problem is based in nerve damage in the cervical spine, osteopathic or chiropractic manipulation may be helpful. In severe cases of disc damage, surgery may be necessary,[143] although the success rate of cervical spine surgery for whiplash injuries is very low.[1]

Most cases of dizziness, however, may simply be an issue of myofascial damage. Thus direct work on the affected structures seems the best solution. Teasell and McCain[145] state that vertigo "generally disappears as painless neck range of motion is restored."

Fattori et al[214] tested the effectiveness of acupuncture on balance disorders after whiplash injury, and found that it was more effective than drugs and physiotherapy.

Proprioceptive disturbance, or vertigo originating in the cervical spine, requires more specific treatment. Loudon et al[272] state that, "Rehabilitation after whiplash injury should focus not only on range of motion and strength but on postural awareness."

Tjell and Rosenhall[350] have reported on the effectiveness of using the Smooth Pursuit Neck Torsion test in the diagnosis of proprioceptive disturbance after whiplash.

In their study, the only subjects that showed indications of cervical proprioceptive interference were the whiplash patients. The authors conclude that this proprioceptive interference may be caused by damage to the facet joints of the cervical spine—just as other researchers have recently concluded (see Neck Pain).

Also, the SPNT test may be a good objective test to provide evidence of whiplash injury:

> "Neck torsion had no effect in subjects with brain stem or vestibular disorders, or an intact balance system, unlike that in patients with WAD [whiplash-associated disorder] with dizziness and, to a lesser extent, in patients with WAD without dizziness. The SPNT test therefore seems to be useful for diagnosing cervical dizziness, at least in patients with WAD having symptoms of dizziness, because it has a high sensitivity and specificity."[350]

Cervical Trauma and Tremor

Ellis[210] details the findings from six cases of patients who developed movement disorders after motor vehicle-induced cervical trauma. The following case—Case 2—is particularly interesting:

> "A 24-year old secretary was sitting in her stationary car when it was hit from behind. She was thrown forwards, restrained by her seat belt, and hit the back of her head against the head rest. Within an hour she had developed a pain in the neck radiating into both arms, associated with paraesthesiae in both arms, but predominantly in the right C5 and C6 distribution. Two weeks after the trauma she developed a tremor in her right hand, particularly on performing activities. She could no longer carry a full cup of coffee and had difficulty holding pen or paper. The neck pain settled to become only intermittent, but the tremor persists 12 months after the accident. Before the trauma she had a very minor tremor, of a different character, present in both hands when under stress.

> "Examination showed mild restriction of neck movements by pain and spasm in the trapeziae, worse on the right. Tone in the limbs was normal. There was slight weakness of hand grip and opponens pollicis on the right. Pin prick sensation was reduced in a C6 distribution in the hand. There was a 6-8 Hz action type tremor, particularly present when the right wrist was extended or flexed and also when the thumb was flexed.

> "Plain cervical spine radiography showed loss of the normal curvature and MRI of the spine was normal."[210]

The C6 distribution of symptoms is interesting, as most of the recent studies on whiplash show that this area of the cervical spine is most susceptible to trauma.

The author reported evidence of nerve root damage or spinal cord involvement in 4 of the six cases. Also, five of the six cases in this report were women, who are more likely to suffer from whiplash injury then men: "Idiopathic torsion dystonia and peripheral induced dystonia are reported to have a female preponderance[249]…This may reflect the higher incidence of joint laxity in the female population[263] with a greater degree of flexion extension resulting from this type of injury."

The author also refers to Jankovic,[249] who suggested criteria for determining whether movement disorders are trauma-related or not. These are:

- Injury must have been severe enough to cause local symptoms for two weeks.
- The onset of the movement disorder should be within a year of the injury.
- The movement disorder must have an anatomical association with the site of the injury.

Systemic Sclerosis and Trauma

Progressive systemic sclerosis (SSc), or scleroderma, is described as, "A chronic disease of unknown cause, characterized by diffuse fibrosis; degenerative changes; and vascular abnormalities in the skin, articular structures, and internal organs (especially the esophagus, intestinal tract, lung, heart, and kidney)." [146]

In this study,[174] the authors describe five case studies of patients who developed SSc after physical trauma. Two of the five were in whiplash accidents. The first patient, a 47-year-old woman, developed symptoms of SSc within a month of her injury; the second patient, a 40-year-old woman, developed her condition 8 weeks after her accident.

"Our observations of the development or exacerbation of SSc following different forms of trauma raise the possibility that trauma can be associated with the onset or an exacerbation of the disease in a small minority of patients. Any causative link must clearly be complex. If a link between trauma and SSc does exist, it seems likely that this simply advances the course of the disease rather than being fundamentally responsible for its development."

Visual Symptoms

Visual symptoms are a well-recognized symptom of whiplash injury. Radanov[119] found the frequency of blurred vision to be 36% in his group of patients. Bogduk[11] reported visual symptoms in 35%. Burke et al[14] performed thorough opthamological examinations on 39 whiplash patients and found that 26.5% had both signs and symptoms of ocular trauma. The most common ocular symptom is blurred vision.[119]

Etiology

Horner's syndrome, or trauma to the cervical sympathetic chain, is a a recognized source of visual disturbances, including blurred vision. The cervical sympathetic chain can be injured during severe hyperextension injuries.[37]

While the occurrence of visual disturbances after whiplash has been documented, little has been studied on the specific etiology of eye damage. Burke et al[14] state, "All but one patient's symptoms were due to ocular motor abnormalities." Such findings could be the result of mild traumatic brain injury, or they could also result from injury to the Posture Control System (see Neck Pain).

Haslett et al[59] have recently identified damage to the retinal blood vessels as another source of eye problems after whiplash. The authors indicate that some of these problems may last for years. They suggest that seatbelt usage increases the forces placed on the delicate structures of the eye, subjecting them to a greater risk of injury.

Prognosis and Treatment

Most cases of visual disturbance heal without invasive therapy, but it may take time. Burke et al[14] found that 70% of patients with visual symptoms were still symptomatic at eight weeks post-trauma, and that 20% of the patients still had problems 12 months after the injury.

The eyes and surrounding musculature are also susceptible to the influence of myofascial tension in the head and neck. Often, release of this tension, especially in the suboccipital muscles, can relieve ocular symptoms.

Symptoms that are severe or that do not show improvement should be referred to an opthamologist.

Sleep Disturbances

Sleep problems as a result of whiplash are fairly common. Radanov et al[119] reported a rate of 69% in one group of whiplash patients.

The most common sleep problems are insomnia and frequent waking. These can be particularly difficult for the patient's recovery, since lack of sleep can lead to fatigue and more pain.

Some patients report increased sleep and a need for daytime naps.

Origins

There seem to be four primary explanations for sleep disturbances after whiplash.

1. Pain itself is probably the most common source of sleep disturbance. Patients in pain simply can't sleep well.
2. Emotional distress, such as anxiety or depression, can result in insomnia.
3. Medication usage can cause sleep problems
4. Post-concussion syndrome, with damage to the brain tissue can result in sleep disturbance.

Treatment

Medications are frequently used for symptoms of sleep disturbance, primarily in the form of benzodiazepines (such as Valium or Xanax.)

Treatment of the somatic pain should be the first priority, and usually sleep disturbances will disappear.

Chapter Three
Prognosis

One of the most common claims made by insurance companies is that whiplash injuries heal within six weeks and that care after that time is unnecessary. While many patients do recover within this six week time period, many studies show that between 20 to 30% of patients have symptoms that last a year or more. The following is a review of these studies.

Prognosis

A number of studies have examined the long-term outcome of whiplash injuries, and the results have been fairly consistent.

Still, Gay and Abbott took these cases seriously, as they state, "We were impressed in our experience with these patients by the importance of preventing accidents that commonly cause whiplash injury of the neck. The symptoms from this condition were so tenacious and the rate of recovery so slow that it was felt that every effort should be made by public authorities to prevent this kind of suffering."

The first study to examine the long-term consequences of whiplash was that done by MacNab[91] in 1964. This study followed up 575 whiplash patients, but he could only review 145 personally. Of these 145, 121 (83%) still had symptoms. MacNab was generous, and assumed that all the unexamined patients had recovered, and concluded, "45 per cent of patients reviewed continued to have some symptoms two years or more after settlement of court action."

Deans et al[26] found that 22.6% of whiplash patients had pain one year after the injury.

Radanov et al[318] found that in a group of whiplash patients, 44% had pain at 3 months, 30% at 6 months, 24% at 12 months, and 18% at 2 years. Only 4% of the patients were considered disabled at two years.

Landy,[261] in an attempt to discredit the notion of long-term whiplash pain wrote, "In conclusion, while 70% of minor head and neck injuries settle within a few weeks of a motor vehicle accident, about 30% continue to complain of headaches and/or neck pain."

Hagstrom and Carlsson[236] found that 13 months after whiplash, "All patients had pain in the neck, 17-33% had headache and 6-17% had pain in various regions of the arms. Thirteen patients (43%) suffered from constant pain, while 17 (57%) had pain-free periods."

Maimaris et al[93] studied 102 patients and found "one-third of all patients with whiplash injuries were still symptomatic 2 years after the accident."

Borchgrevnick et al,[184] on the other hand, found that after 2½ years, 58% of their whiplash patients reported symptoms from their collision. Women were more likely to have symptoms at follow-up than men, and had significantly higher reports of neck pain, dizziness, and nausea than men who reported symptoms.

Bylund and Bjornstig[194] reported on a four year study of 255 people in car accidents. Rear-end collisions were responsible for only 39% of the injuries. However, 64% of the sick leave used within 2.5 years of the collision was by people in rear-end collisions, and at the four-year follow-up, 89% of those on disability had been in rear-end collisions. Only 8% of the occupants in rear-end collisions were receiving disability payments 4 to 6 years after their accidents.

One study by Gargan and Bannister examined patients an average of 10.8 years after the accident and found that only 12% had recovered completely.[48] A 1994 study by the same authors[47] found that 48% of whiplash patients had symptoms one year after their injury, but that this increased to 62% at a two year follow-up. At the 15-year follow-up[341] they found that of the 40 patients available for study, 28 (70%) continued to report pain

Between 20 and 30% of people in rear end collisions suffer long-term pain.

from their injury. "Symptoms had remained static in 54%, improved in 18%, and deteriorated in 28%. All patients who had been involved in litigation had settled an average of 14 years earlier than this study, so litigation played no role in these symptoms. The study also reported that 80% of those patients who had deteriorated had radiological evidence of degenerative changes. Patients at higher risk for long-term symptoms were those who were older, and who had radiating pain from their injuries. Psychological distress was detected in 52% of the patients with symptoms.

Capistrant,[15] writing about thoracic outlet syndrome as a sequela of whiplash, had sixteen patients with symptoms after an average of 29 months after the original injury. He also reported objective findings of nerve conduction loss that demonstrated that the pain was not fabricated.

Radanov et al[123] found that at six months after the accident, 19% of patients still had headache symptoms related to the injury.

Radanov et al[119] examined 117 whiplash patients in regard to psychological status. The researchers focused on reported well-being, cognitive ability, and personality traits, to see if abnormal ratings on any of these scales corresponded to long-term disability. "In summary, the results indicated that: (1) the disposition of patients (personality traits) does not primarily influence the course of recovery from common whiplash; (2) psychological and cognitive problems of patients with common whiplash may rather be seen as correlates of somatic symptoms." The authors conclude that the psychological distress seen in many chronic whiplash patients is not proof of malingering, but, on the contrary, these symptoms result from chronic pain.

Parmar and Raymakers[112] found that 18% of whiplash patients had "significant pain" two years after the injury. This was also substantiated by Murray et al.[295]

Hodgson and Grundy[65] reviewed forty patients, 26 of with whiplash injuries, and 14 with neck pain from side or front impact accidents. All patients had been involved in compensation. The patients were reviewed between 10 and 15 years after the injury, and the researchers found that 62% of the whiplash patients had residual symptoms, while only 14% of the other patients did.

Hildingsson and Toolanen[64] studied 93 accident victims, 45 of whom were in rear-end collisions. "At follow-up, on an average of 2 years after the accident, 42 percent had recovered completely, 15 percent had minor discomfort, and 43 percent had discomfort sufficient to interfere with their capacity for work."

Evans[37] wrote that there are certain symptoms of whiplash that are more likely to result in long-term disability. "Risk factors for a less favorable prognosis include the presence of intrascapular or upper back pain, occipital headache, multiple symptoms or paresthesias at presentation, reduced range of movement of the cervical spine, the presence of an objective neurologic deficit, and preexisting degenerative osteoarthritic changes."

An editorial by Carette[16] in the *New England Journal of Medicine* sums up the current thinking on whiplash: "Although the majority [of whiplash patients] become asymptomatic in a matter of weeks to a few months, 20 to 40 percent have symptoms that are sometimes debilitating and persist for years...The reality is that some patients with a whiplash injury do not recover completely."

The Quebec Task Force

The Quebec Task Force has been used by some to claim that whiplash injuries are only short-term problems and that whiplash patients should be completely recovered within a few weeks. Freeman and Croft,[219] however, wrote about the serious flaws with the Task Force findings:

"The validity of the conclusions and recommendations of the Quebec Task Force regarding the natural course of whiplash injuries is questionable. This lack of validity stems from the presence of bias, the use of unconventional terminology, and conclusions that are not concurrent with the literature the Task Force accepted for review. Although the Quebec Task Force set out to 'redefine whiplash and its management,' striving for the desirable goal of clarification of the numerous contentious issues surrounding the injury, its publications instead have confused the subject further."

Certain factors can predict long-term disability.

Delayed Onset

Often it is the case that insurance companies will attempt to discredit a patient's whiplash symptoms by saying that the patient did not report any symptoms at the time of the accident. The insurance companies say that these patients are malingering.

The scientific evidence does not support these claims. On the contrary, the medical literature is full of evidence that the symptoms of whiplash do not necessarily begin at the time of the accident.

Schutt and Dohan[132] also found that delayed onset of symptoms, "was not associated with longer duration of disability."

Teasell and McCain[145] wrote, "A delay in symptoms of several hours is characteristic of whiplash injuries. Most patients feel little or no pain for the first few hours following the injury, after which symptoms gradually intensify. During this time period findings on examination are generally minimal.."

Hagstrom and Carlsson[236] found that in 30 whiplash patients, pain appeared on the day of the accident in 24 of the patients. "The other 6 patients reported a pain-free interval from the accident of varying length; in 4 patients the delay exceeded 3 months."

Wolff's Headache[157] states, "The physical examination is usually normal during the initial 2 to 3 hours following neck trauma. However, after this initial period, anterior neck swelling and tenderness may be observed, particularly in acceleration-extension injuries, thus restricting neck movement."

Weiss et al[153] on posttraumatic migraine wrote, "The headaches began within hours to days of the injury." One of the patients in this study, who suffered a whiplash injury in which there "was no direct head trauma or loss of consciousness," reported numbness in her arms immediately after the accident, but did not have any headaches until several days after the injury.

In regard to ocular symptoms, Burke et al[14] report that one "patient first noted signs and symptoms of convergence and accommodative insufficiency some 10 days after the accident."

Ettlin et al,[36] in their study of cerebral symptoms after whiplash found a delay of up to three days in the onset of concentration problems.

Evans,[38] on post-concussion syndrome states, "The time interval from the injury to the first onset of migraine can vary from a few hours to weeks."

Capistrant[15] found that in a group of 35 thoracic outlet syndrome patients, "In 20 cases, there was an average delay of 5 months between cervical strain injury and arm symptoms."

Some symptoms take days or weeks to develop after an accident.

Chapter Four
Controversies

Mild Traumatic Brain Injury and Post-Concussion Syndrome

The fragility of the brain has been recognized for centuries. Gama, in 1835, wrote, "Fibers as delicate as those of which the organ of mind is composed are liable to break as a result of violence to the head." [38]

Mild traumatic brain injury is a major problem in our society. Ruff et al[329] wrote this about the extent of the problem:

> "Epidemiological evidence suggests that each year in the United States alone, over 1,300,000 individuals suffer MTBI. Ongoing studies at New York University further suggest that, after 1 year, about 10% of their MTBI sample continues to complain of post-concussional symptoms, and about 11% of those who were previously employed have not returned to work. Thus, if even a small proportion (10%) present with persistent problems, over 130,000 individuals are affected each year in the United States. Thus, the Miserable Minority represents a sizable challenge to the health-care system."

There is a tremendous amount of confusion, controversy, and misinformation on the issue of (MTBI), post-concussion syndrome (PCS), and whiplash injuries.

On one side of the equation are physicians who believe that the Postconcussion Syndrome (PCS) is faked. In fact, in a recent survey[39] of physicians attitudes about PCS and whiplash, nearly 25% of family practice doctors and 23% of orthopedists reported that they questioned the authenticity of PCS. They were even more likely to question the validity of whiplash.

On the other side is another group of physicians that strongly believe that the psychiatric and attentional difficulties after whiplash are a result of neurological damage to the brain.

Complicating the whole issue is the role of chronic pain. Pain as a result of tissue damage can also overlap with the symptoms found in patients with MTBI.[120,318,329,335,346,359]

Kessels et al[253] studied a group of 24 whiplash patients in regard to this issue, with no definitive answer. They surmised that the patients' distress could, "...be related to both emotional distress caused by the accident itself and to additional experienced stressing life events, either prior to the accident or during recovery. However, these high scores could also be the consequence of organical lesions, causing physical complaints (e.g. neck pain or headache) that lead to psychological stress."

Packard and Ham wrote that, "...many patients sustaining MHI suffer from significant difficulties with concentration, memory, and/or thinking. The ability to concentrate and remember important details is often a major factor in determining an individual's ability to function in society. Sometimes these symptoms may be overlooked or disbelieved because of a 'minor' injury, no car damage, low velocity impact, and so forth. There also may be a prejudice against these patients because of legal proceedings or physician and attorney bias. Cognitive deficits may only be evident when an individual is under a great deal of stress, overtired, or trying to do more than one thing at a time. We have found that many patients are only aware of cognitive difficulty under these circumstances or when attempting to return to work or increase their activity level. These difficulties may be compounded when patients are evaluated with head imaging studies (CT or MRI) that are 'normal.' Unfortunately, a 'normal' imaging study is often considered to mean normal function."[306]

Etiology

As we saw in the section on Biomechanics, tremendous forces can be applied to the body during a "mild" whiplash accident.

Parker and Rosenblum[307] provide a thorough summary of the causes of MTBI:

"TBI needs only sufficient angular rotation (without impact) to occur, although unreported head impact in MVA is common. Rear-end impact causes the head on the relaxed neck to be left behind momentarily. Front-end collision causes the head to be propelled forward. The head moves in a combination of planes (lateral and sagittal) and torsion around the tethering neck, which changes the brain's position and movement relative to the enclosing skull and often causes impact within the confining space. It is unpredictable which structures will be over-stressed and damaged. TBI is determined by: the point of impact and its direction, velocity, and accelerating or decelerating effect; whether the neck is braced; whether the rotation is accelerated or steady; the relative strength of the head-neck junction; ratio of brain mass to head mass; duration of the impact impulse; and characteristics of the scalp. Intensive head movement causes contusions of the frontal and temporal poles from *translational* motion, most severe at the crests of gyri, but which can extend subcortically. Lacerations occur of the base of the brain from *lateral* or angular motion. *Rotation* in the coronal plane causes shearing of internal structures and penetrating blood vessels and tensile and compression strains. Head impact causes skull and brain deformation; energy directed inwardly coup, contre-coup and/or diffuse brain injury, and pressure gradients."

Friedmann et al[45] wrote, "Patients receiving whiplash injury of the neck can also suffer from a cerebral concussion. If the head is thrown forward and then strikes the steering wheel or windshield, a head injury can occur. Also, mechanical deformation of the brain occurs during the acceleration/deceleration phase of the injury and a concussion can occur without the head actually striking anything."

Teasell and McCain[145] elaborate: "It has been proposed that rotational brain shear injuries occur as a result of sudden movement of the skull, especially sudden angular acceleration, resulting in surface trauma to the cerebral cortex and cerebellum. This theory posits that the brain lies relatively free within the skull. As the head moves, the brain, because of its inertia, tends to maintain its position within the vault. The moving skull may therefore concuss the brain either as it rotates backward or as it accelerates forward."

Research by Otte et al[303,304,305] have used the much more sensitive PET and SPECT scans on whiplash patients, and have found evidence of brain dysfunction. In one study, they wrote:

"[Our] hypothesis is that parieto-occipital hypometabolism may be caused by activation of nociceptive afferences from the upper cervical spine. By contrast, the areas of hypometabolism seen in areas other than parieto-occipital may mainly be explained by brain contusion and not by the effects of activated nociceptive afferences on brain metabolism. In addition, hypometabolism in parieto-occipital regions cannot be excluded in some cases as part or entirely a consequence of diffuse axonal lesions due to acceleration forces."[303]

In a later study,[304] they elaborate on this issue. The authors hypothesized that if head trauma was responsible for the cerebral lesions, they should only exist in one of two areas—the left frontal and the right parieto-occipital regions. They did indeed find lesions in these areas. They also, however, found areas of hypoperfusion in the left parieto-occipital region.

> "As the patients were looking to the right side at the time of the accident, a contusion mechanism could be possible for the left frontal and the right parieto-occipital region, regardless of whether this was produced directly by hitting the head onto the steering wheel or by the acceleration forces producing indirect head impact. If whiplash injury were only a form of mild head injury with a contusion mechanism, the additional left parieto-occipital hypoperfusion in the above patients could not be explained. Therefore, we think that parieto-occipital hypoperfusion in whiplash patients may still be hypothesized to be elicited from lesions of neuroceptive afferents from the cervical spine. Of course, this does not mean that brain contusions need not be carefully evaluated, as additional contusion is well known to have an effect on clinical after injury."[304]

Torres and Shapiro[148] tested this theory by giving whiplash patients electroencephalogram (EEG) tests. They found that 46% of these patients showed abnormal EEG readings. Abnormal EEGs after whiplash have also been found by Jacome et al[70] and Ettlin et al.[36]

Ommaya,[109] in simulated whiplash with monkeys, found that non-contact injuries can result in cerebral concussion and bleeding on the surface of the brain and upper spinal cord. Ommaya and Yarnell[108] also found subdural hematomas in two whiplash patients.

Viktrup et al[354] reported on a case of man who died of stroke after a whiplash injury. The stroke was caused by injury to the vertebral artery (See Neck Pain).

Does Concussion Require Loss of Consciousness?

Many professionals mistakenly believe that concussion requires a loss of consciousness. A number of studies have dealt with this misconception. Kelly and Rosenberg[252] provide a thorough summation of this literature:

> "Concussion is a trauma-induced alteration in mental status that may or may not involve loss of consciousness. The misunderstanding that concussion requires loss of consciousness has surfaced again in recent years. More than 30 years ago, the Congress of Neurological Surgeons[322] concluded that head injury leading to mental status alterations without loss of consciousness is also a form of concussion. C. Miller Fisher[215] also offered a clear case of amnesia from head injury without loss of consciousness, and he alluded to numerous other reports in his experience and in the literature of similar cases. Ommaya and Gennarelli[299] created an animal model of traumatic brain injury in which three of the six grades of concussion did not involve loss of consciousness. More recent animal studies[314] also found axonal swelling after mild traumatic brain injury in animals, further demonstrating that neuroanatomic alterations indeed occur during concussion."

Symptoms

The symptoms of post-concussion syndrome can be difficult to separate from the common symptoms of whiplash. The following is a listing of symptoms that may be a result of PCS.

Headache. Evans[37] states, "Because head injuries are commonly associated with neck trauma, the headaches may be perpetuated by neck pathology such as myofascial injury, vertebral disk disease, or exacerbation of preexisting spondolysis." But headaches need not be soft-tissue related. Matthews[94] described the condition he called "footballer's migraine," or migraine headaches in young men with mild head trauma from playing soccer. Similar kinds of headache have been reported from boxing, American football, and rugby. Ommaya and Yarnell's patients both reported headaches.[108]

Dizziness is a common symptom of mild head injury, although other factors can be responsible (see Dizziness section).[38]

Hearing loss can result from head injury, either from blood in the middle ear, disruption of the ossicular chain, or damage to the brain. Hearing loss is a serious symptom, and a referral is imperative.[38]

Psychological symptoms. MTBI can be devastating to those who suffer from it, and psychological symptoms are very common after such injuries. Cicerone and Kalmar[202] addressed the common misconception that pre-existing depression is at the root of Post-concussion syndrome. They found no differences between depressed and non-depressed patients.

Machulda et al,[276] however, found that patients with pre-existing, but subclinical, psychological symptoms experienced an exacerbation of those symptoms after MTBI. They found that it was not the number of stressful events in the subjects' lives that resulted in increased symptoms, but how that individual responded to the stressful events:

> "Our results are also consistent with an emerging literature on postconcussive syndrome, which proposes that pre-existing characterological features that are subclinical and do not differentiate individuals under stable, nonstressful conditions come to the forefront under stressful situations...In other words, normal variance in individuals' response to stress in most environmental conditions is exaggerated when they are faced with more challenging, and often confusing, environmental conditions, such as mild traumatic brain injury."

Visual symptoms such as blurred vision, are also fairly common from whiplash injuries. These symptoms can also result from damage to the brain, and the patient should be referred to rule out serious pathology.[38]

Smell and taste are two other sensations that can be damaged by mild head trauma. If a patient reports disturbance in either of these, a referral is necessary.[38]

Cognitive dysfunction is a well-documented symptom of whiplash injuries.[120,122] Ettlin et al[36] found that of 21 patients with acute whiplash, 13 had concentration deficits. Other brain functions that can be disturbed include "information processing speed, attention, reaction time, and memory for new information." [36] Perlis wrote, "Microlesions from twisting and shearing may damage structures associated with both arousal and sleep generation."[310]

Sleep disturbances, fatigue, lethargy, or drowsiness can also be caused by brain injury, but they may also be caused by general pain from the injury as well.[38]

Other symptoms that can be the result of concussion are mania, seizures (rare), amnesia (rare), and movement disorders (rare).[38]

Warning Signs

If in doubt about a patient's symptoms, make a referral to someone qualified to diagnose the problem. As we've seen, most of the problems associated with whiplash are not life-threatening. With head injuries, though, a symptom that seems benign may not be. The following is a short list of warning signs of possible serious brain damage:[36,38,120,122,383]

- Did the patient hit her or his head in the accident?
- Did the patient lose consciousness in the accident?
- Did the patient report amnesia?
- Is the patient confused? Check with other caregivers, family, friends of the patient to see if there has been a change in cognitive functioning after the accident.
- Is the patient forgetful? Does he or she show up late or miss appointments? While there may be many reasons for forgetting important appointments, this may be a symptom of concussion.
- Has the patient noticed any movement problems? Has the client become "clumsy?"
- Has the patient reported an increased sensitivity to noise or light?

- Is the patient have a history of alcoholism or drug abuse? Evans[38] states, "An increased number of posttraumatic sequelae and additional slowing of reaction time are associated with a history of prior alcohol abuse. Alcohol intoxication makes the initial assessment of patients with head injury more difficult and is a risk factor for neurosurgical sequelae."
- Does the patient report pronounced lethargy, sleepiness, or drowsiness?

Parker[308] provided the additional reactions that he found in a group of 33 MTBI patients:

- Persistent altered consciousness: feelings of discomfort in one's body, dissociation, and being in a "fog."
- Cerebral personality disorder:
  - A reduced intensity of feelings, apathy, depression, indifference.
  - Aprosodia, or a lack of "expressive movements which serve communications and regulate social relationships" (i.e. facial responses, prosody of speech (e.g., deficits of pitch, loudness, timbre, tempo, stress, accent)).
  - Irritability, violence, anger, anxiety.
  - Personality change. "A young woman was in a car that was rear-ended at high speed. She experienced retrograde amnesia for 15 minutes and post-traumatic amnesia for 10 minutes. Initially she complained only of neck injuries. No positive findings were determined at the ER. She had been friendly, wanted to continue her education, was able to work 6½ hours a day at a bank, had normal habits, and no urge to gamble. A month later her personality changed. She always wanted to go out. She started to gamble once a month, then every 2 weeks, every weekend, and ultimately staying overnight. She would buy things...and give them away without apparent reason. In order to obtain money for gambling, she stole cash from [her job] which, with her paycheque she lost through gambling. When asked what she expected, she thought she would win enough to be able to return it."
- Thirty-one of the 33 patients were found to have a second psychiatric diagnosis in addition to brain trauma. These were most often depression (12 of 33, or 36%) and PTSD (16 of 33, or 48%).
- The patients who met diagnostic criteria for PTSD expressed anxiety, suspiciousness, fear of accidents and attack, nightmares, and a preoccupation with thoughts of the accident.
- Other symptoms discovered included excessive alcohol use, denial of disability, and sexual dysfunction.

An additional risk factor for head injury is the use of the drug warfarin, an anticoagulant. Volans[355] witnessed three cases of severe intracranial bleeding after MTBI in patients using the drug. Volans suggests the following guidelines:

1. All head injury patients should be questioned for warfarin use—especially if over 60 years old.
2. All head injury patients taking warfarin should have a measure of their anticoagulation.
3. Any patient that has abnormally decreased coagulation should have it controlled.
4. If there are signs of neurological symptoms, specifically headache complaints, patient should undergo a CT.
5. If abnormalities appear on CT, patient may need immediate reversal of anticoagulation to prevent further deterioration.

Even if the patient has well-controlled coagulation and no other obvious symptoms, **they are still at risk**. It is strongly advised to perform a CT scan to check for possible hemorrhaging.

A combination of any of these risk factors and symptoms may warrant a referral to a neuropsychological specialist.

Diagnosis

The Importance of A Careful Review

Andary et al[173] wrote, "We propose that the [chronic pain] patients who endorse or complain of memory or concentration problems, who express confusion about their diagnosis, complain of pain in head, neck, and arms, and/or were injured in motor vehicle accident should be further questioned about the possibility of concurrent TBI."

There is evidence that MTBI is often times missed by physicians. Moss and Wade[294] examined the medical records of 107 hospital admissions to a trauma ward, looking specifically for undiagnosed head injury. Of the 107 patients, 47 had a head injury—but 24 of these were not diagnosed. Those patients most likely to be overlooked were those with "mild or trivial injuries," in which 66% of the diagnoses were missed.

That head injury from "minor" whiplash accidents can easily be overlooked is evident from two severe cases cited in this study: "One patient jumped from a five-storey building, sustaining many severe injuries, including a laceration to the forehead but *the notes did not record any head injury*. A second patient fell 3000 feet with a partially opened parachute: the main injury noted was of the back, but there had been some bleeding from the nose, and later notes recorded bruising developing around one eye; again, *there was no diagnosis of a head injury in the medical notes*." [Emphasis added.][294]

The authors stress the importance of posttraumatic amnesia (PTA) in trauma cases. Patients with PTA may not report head injury at the time of hospital treatment, simply because they don't remember the injury. "...PTA may easily be missed in a busy casualty department especially when other injuries dominate immediate treatment needs."[294]

Often, an ER doctor is not looking for MTBI, but for more serious trauma. When the physician sees that "nothing is wrong," the patient is released.

The diagnosis of MTBI when it doesn't exist can also lead to problems. Taylor et al[346] warn that a misdiagnosis of "brain damage" can "lead to unnecessary lifelong suffering."

Imaging

Persistent Post-Concussion Syndrome (PPCS) is one of the most frustrating conditions to work with, simply because most imaging studies are not powerful enough to detect subtle brain tissue damage; MRI and CT scans usually show nothing in patients with long-term symptoms.

Moore[292] discusses the problem of MRI scans: "Currently there are no studies showing that symptoms correlate with neuroimaging abnormalities or vice versa. Conversely, a normal MRI scan does not exclude serious neurologic injury. In 24 of 434 *fatal* non-missile head injuries, the only abnormality was microscopic diffuse axonal injury — these lesions would *not be detected by MRI*."

Karlsborg et al[251] reported that in two whiplash patients, "small punctate areas of increased signal intensity on T2-weighted and protodensity images were found in the occipital lobes suggesting petecchial hemorrhage; however, both patients had normal MRI at follow-up 7 months later."

SPECT scans show promise in this arena. Researchers have found evidence of brain lesions in whiplash patients. Now some new research has been published that adds substantially to this work.[305,374]

Kant et al[250] investigated 43 patients with "persistent post-concussion syndrome"—or patients with symptoms of PCS an average of 477 days since their injury. All of the patients had mild closed head injury: 47% from motor vehicle accidents; 19% from falls; and 30% from assaults or a falling object. Thirty-nine of these patients had been given an MRI scan, and 21 had been given a CT scan before this study began.

The researchers performed a SPECT scan on each patient, and then compared abnormal findings on this series to findings on MRI and CT.

Of the 43 patients, SPECT found abnormalities in 23 (53%) of the subjects. MRI found abnormalities in just 3 patients, and CT in only two patients. The authors found that, in all, 22 patients (51%) had evidence of brain tissue damage on SPECT that was not detected by other imaging methods.

Tests

A new line of research may hold some promise. A number of studies have reported finding high levels of protein S-100 in patients with intracranial disease or injury. "The protein is synthesized in astroglial cells in all parts of the CNS. It is normally not detectable in serum, while high serum levels indicate damage to glial cells and blood-brain barrier dysfunction." [361]

Computerized tests found that patients with elevated S-100 had a significantly slower response time, as well as more difficulty with attention.

While the study group was small, the authors cautiously conclude, "The present results may indicate that the presence of protein S-100 is a useful predictive and prognostic biochemical serum marker for persistent neurocognitive dysfunction after MHI." [361]

Packard and Ham[306] reported that EEG exams may have some validity in determining the role of brain injury and headache after whiplash.

Treatment

It is important for the patient to understand the nature of the condition. Evans[38] states, "Many patients are greatly reassured to discover that their symptoms are not unique or crazy but are instead part of a well-described syndrome."

It is also critical that patients with suspected MTBI get referred to a neuropsychologist so that appropriate diagnosis and treatment can be determined.

Course of Recovery

Silver and McAllister[383] wrote, "For most patients, recovery is rapid, with difficulties receding over the subsequent weeks to months. In general, the prognosis is favorable for complete recovery 6 to 12 months after the injury. A small but significant percentage will have persistent signs and symptoms of varying severity on a chronic basis. Some will suffer a single symptom such as headache." [383]

Both the psychological and physical aspects of MTBI must be addressed. McClelland[288] wrote, "A current model of postconcussion syndrome is that the early and possibly the middle phases (i.e., the period up to about 12 weeks post injury) are the direct result of brain injury, while the persistent (late phase) is a secondary psychological reaction."

Most patients recover from head injury in 6 to 12 months.

Psychology of MTBI

Ruff et al[329] describes the importance of determining the existence of psychological problems before the injury, so that an accurate assessment of the trauma can be determined. They found that the effects of MTBI can interact with personality factors and a past history of trauma to make recovery slow and difficult. For instance, patients who are used to being in total control may feel that they now have none, and may try to dictate treatment. Or patients who are perfectionists before their trauma may be severely depressed when they can no longer sustain their perfection.

One of the patients in this study was a college student who used her ability in college to bury an unhappy past. After her mild head injury, this facade started to fall apart, and she became suicidal.

All of the patients in this series had a documented head injury (one from whiplash), but concurrent psychological issues made treatment much more complicated. "As adults these individuals developed psychological defenses which enabled them to have some of their previously frustrated needs met, which preserved a sense of self-esteem. However, their prior needs and insecurities were reactivated by the MTBI."

"MTBI can cause a significant breakdown in psychological defenses and character style in at least two ways: first, defenses can be damaged by brain injury itself; secondly, the breakdown of defenses can occur as a reaction to relating with professionals, friends, colleagues, and family members." [329]

"It is crucial to recognize the extent to which the initial breakdown in defenses has resulted directly from brain-based alterations caused by the trauma. TBI individuals may no longer think as efficiently or logically as before..." Furthermore, "It is not an uncommon experience for individuals with MTBI to have their symptoms questioned and, not infrequently, dismissed."

Helping these patients is even more difficult when one tries to find out about preexisting psychological issues. As the authors write, "One of the ironies of forensic evaluations is that premorbid emotional dysfunctioning may be identified and explored for the primary purpose of dismissing the significance of the MTBI, rather than achieving a case formulation that integrates organic and non-organic factors."[329] Questioning patients about psychological issues pre-injury, if not done carefully, can make the patient afraid that you are questioning the validity of his or her condition.

Drugs

Petterson and Toolanen[312] recently examined the role of methylprednisolone in the prevention of chronic whiplash pain.

"Methylprednisolone has shown neuroprotective and potent anti-inflammatory effects. In patients with spinal cord injuries methylprednisolone, administered within 8 hours after the trauma, improved recovery and had a neuroprotective effect."

The drug also has analgesic properties, and serious side effects—including peptic ulcers, psychic stimulation, and the drug's long period of effect. Its use in this study, however, is revealing in regard to whiplash. The researchers stated that they "strictly" followed the same administration procedure of the drug as previously and regularly used in spinal cord injury cases. The motivation for trying this kind of therapy was explained:

"The hypothesis is that chronic symptoms after whiplash injury are not only of musculoskeletal origin, but also could emanate from the central nervous system. Thus, patients with multiple symptoms, including persistent neck pain, dizziness, paresthesia, and cognitive impairment, may have a lesion of the central nervous system, contrary to monosymptomatic patients with intermittent neck pain."

The study was a small one, but the authors found that the methylprednisolone patients had fewer symptoms at the six-month follow-up and had used significantly few sick days than the placebo group.

Major damage to the brain may require surgical intervention, although this is rare after whiplash injuries. A patient that has been diagnosed with post-concussion syndrome is likely to be given medications — primarily antidepressants and antianxiety drugs.[38] Other drugs may be given for headache.

Psychological Symptoms

Whiplash can be a very distressing event, and symptoms of emotional distress are common.[118] Radanov et al[119] reported that 55% of one group of whiplash patients suffered from anxiety. Mayou et al[95] reported that 41% of whiplash patients in their study "reported anxiety or depression above the usually accepted thresholds for clinical disorder."

Smed et al[337] wrote, "Pain in the neck, which accompanies all whiplash injuries, certainly interferes with daily activities, reminding the sufferer of the accident at every movement."

Types of Problems

Anxiety and phobia related to driving in a car are common symptoms of whiplash. Mayou et al[95] found that one year after the accident, 22% of whiplash patients still had major concerns about driving, and 38% still had minor concerns. If these symptoms are severe, the patient may be suffering from Post Traumatic Stress Disorder. (See PTSD section.)

Depression is also common. It is believed by many to not be a specific problem of whiplash, but rather a general problem of chronic pain. Lee et al[84] stated, "Depression scores, and ratings of whiplash pain...were greatest in patients with long-standing pain." Von Korff and Simon[356] wrote in regard to their study of patients with chronic pain and depression, "[A]s pain became more diffuse, depressive symptoms showed pronounced increments in severity. This result is consistent with a large body of research showing that diffuse somatic symptoms are associated with increased psychological distress."

Shalev et al[380] found that depression was common after trauma, and was often associated with symptoms of PTSD.

Anger is an important symptom to keep in mind when working with whiplash patients. A study by Duckro et al[29] reported that there is a direct relationship between depression, pain, and anger. A study by Chemtob et al[17] found that anger played an important role in PTSD. Hatch et al[60] reported that patients with tension headaches had high levels of suppressed anger.

Mayou[287] elaborates on the importance of addressing anger issues. "Anger is not uncommon in physical illness and is a prominent reaction of many innocent victims of trauma; anger about the suffering, anger towards those responsible, and anger about the lack of recognition of the suffering and disability. Anger influences attitudes to the pursuit of compensation; it is often focused on the lack of concern or apology by those believed to be responsible rather than on gaining maximum financial reward. For example, in medical malpractice, the way in which the complaint is handled is a very important determinant as to whether any litigation is pursued."

Substance abuse is another issue that should be addressed in whiplash patients. Whether pre-existing or a way of coping with chronic pain, substance abuse can seriously undermine rehabilitation.[38] Patients with chronic pain should be evaluated for the possibility of analgesic rebound headache, as well (see Headache).

Etiology

There are a number of causes of psychological symptoms from whiplash injuries:

Undiagnosed or Untreated Pain

This is a common source of emotional distress after whiplash injury.[119] Merskey[99] wrote, "Patients also become depressed, which is scarcely surprising if they have to suffer a number of the foregoing symptoms and are suspected of malingering."

Chronic pain is a difficult problem that has many physicians stymied, as seen in a number of studies. The attitude of some physicians is clearly illustrated by the statement by Encel and Johnston,[167] "Pain may be retained even though there be no adequate physical stimulus for such a pain...Experience leads us to believe that it is real pain, but less real than the pain resulting from a physical disorder affecting the pain endings and thalamic system." The authors don't elaborate on what "less real" means exactly. This determining of real and "less real" pain is completely arbitrary, as shown by another study done by Hendler and Kozikowski.[62]

In this study, 60 chronic pain patients involved with litigation with broad diagnoses such as "chronic pain" or "psychogenic pain" were carefully examined, and two thirds of these patients were found to have real pathology that had been unrecognized, undiagnosed, and untreated by previous physicians. The authors state, "Unfortunately, the psychiatric abnormalities that are the normal response to chronic pain tend to bias physicians, causing them to perform significantly less-extensive evaluations."

Gargan et al[224] studied the relationship between psychological distress and whiplash, and wrote, "Our findings suggest that the symptoms of whiplash injury have both physical and psychological components, and that the psychological response develops after the physical damage. Both physical and behavioral responses to these injuries are established in most cases within three months of injury. This suggests that the greatest potential for influencing the natural history of the syndrome is within this period."

Much of the anger and hostility seen in some patients is directed at medical and legal professionals, who may be seen as the enemy. Kelly[74] wrote, "It is clearly not surprising that people, who, through no fault of their own, have been involved in an accident should feel resentful...This resentment is compounded when they meet disbelief from the medical profession and the lawyers, a refusal to treat their symptoms, and a vague hint of moral disapproval that they should dare seek compensation for their financial loss."

Thus, a pattern of chronic whiplash seems to develop with some patients:

1. A whiplash accident with soft-tissue injury.
2. Patient is thrust into confrontation with the insurance company.
3. Stress from interactions with the insurance company exacerbates the pain symptoms,
4. Resulting in chronic physical and psychological symptoms.

Listening to the patient and taking his or her pain seriously is critical in developing a good working relationship.

Psychological Symptoms Disappear When Physical Pain Treated

The idea that psychological symptoms are a result of untreated pain is further substantiated by Wallis et al.[360] They recently reported that when the physical symptoms of whiplash pain were treated and alleviated, the psychological symtoms vanished immediately. They wrote:

> "[The study results confirm] the notion that psychological distress is secondary to pain than with the belief that somehow all whiplash patients have the same premorbid disposition to a characteristic psychological profile which underlies their complaint of pain. Somatisation, obsessive-compulsive behaviour, and depression can readily be seen as rational psychological responses to persisting pain that medical practitioners have not been able to diagnose or treat, and which has been attributed to malingering. These rational responses should disappear if the underlying pain is successfully treated; this is what occurred in the present study."

The Effect of Chronic Pain

The physical limitations that occur after some whiplash injuries can seriously undermine mental health. Mayou et al[95] found that the severity of psychological symptoms in whiplash patients were related to the amount of number of medical complications. Radanov et al[120] found that the attentional functioning of chronic whiplash patients could be traced to disabling headaches; this group also had more psychological symptoms. Duckro et al[29] state, "The co-occurence of affective disturbance and chronic headache is a common finding in the literature."

Mendelson[97] examined two groups of chronic low back pain patients: one group seeking compensation, and the other not seeking compensation. He found that both groups suffered the same amount of pain and the same number of psychological symptoms. He stated, "... there is no support for the claim that personal injury litigants describe their pain as more severe than do non-litigants..."

More recently, Wallis et al[359] compared whiplash patients to patients with other types of chronic pain and concluded that the psychological profile of patients, "lends itself readily to the interpretation that the psychological distress exhibited by patients with whiplash is secondary to chronic pain."

Differentiating Organic and Psychogenic Pain

Adler et al[169] found the following differences between patients with organic pain (OP) and patients with psychogenic pain (PP):

1. The organic pain group (OP) localized their pain more, while for the psychogenic pain (PP) patients, the pain was more diffuse and vague.
2. The OP group used more sensory rather than affective and evaluative words when describing their pain. "...an example of an 'affective' adjective: *frightening*; and a 'sensory' adjective: *burning*."
3. "The OP group described more discrete changes in pain intensity and in periodicity. The OP group more frequently mentioned pain intensifying factors, and intensifying factors dependent on voluntary movement." The OP patients were also more likely to mention factors that *decreased* their pain than the PP patients.
4. Men in the OP group were more likely to see their pain as a symptom, rather than a disease itself.
5. The OP men more often had intact personal relationships, and "used straightforward, simple language, free of medical jargon" to describe their pain.

Family Support

Whiplash is one of the most difficult injuries in terms of social interactions. There are no obvious injuries (i.e., broken bones, wounds), and so friends, co-workers, and relatives may have a difficult time understanding what the patient is going through. They may even believe that the patient is making it up.

Schwartz et al[129] studied the relationship between chronic pain patients and spouses. They found that patients performing tasks with their spouses present experienced more pain and less endurance than those patients performing without their spouses present. The researchers suggest that some relationships may actually perpetuate pain patterns.

It is important to evaluate the level of family support with whiplash patients. Education aimed at the spouse or relatives can also be an important part in helping a whiplash patient recover.

Pre-Existing Psychological Disorder

Borchgrevink et al[183] reviews the literature which explains the relationship between personality-type and whiplash:

"Common neck sprain injuries (whiplash) are usually caused by car collisions and the characteristics of these injuries are the occurrence of considerable pain and prolonged disability in some patients despite a lack of objective signs of pathology. Many studies have been published to explain this phenomenon. One suggestions is that persisting symptoms after neck sprain injury are caused by neurosis. Hodge[243] even named this condition whiplash neurosis. He claimed that almost all these individuals with prolonged disabilities after neck sprain injury had preexisting personalities with strong elements of hostility and dependency, but he gave no empirical support for his views. Hoffman[66] studied 110 patients, most of them suffering from whiplash syndrome, and claiming for compensation. He found that 89% of the patients suffered from emotional symptoms and 30% from exaggerated personality traits or personality disorders; that is, traits which had been aggravated by the accident. In a prospective study, Yarnell et al[373] found that 8 of 14 whiplash patients had abnormal scores on measures of depression, anxiety, and character disturbance. In contrast, recent prospective studies using less selected and larger samples, have found that psychological and social variables do not predict the persistence of physical symptoms related to the injury at 1-year[285] and 2-year[318] follow-up, although the latter study suggested that the baseline scores of nervousness and spontaneous aggressiveness, as measured by the Freiburg Personality Inventory, were higher for symptomatic compared to asymptomatic patients. Interestingly, a study by Drottning et al[208] found that whiplash patients with higher emotional responses measured only hours after the injury, reported more neck pain 4 weeks later. This finding is consistent with Malt and Olafsen[280] who found that psychological and emotional short time responses were strongly related to preaccidental life circumstances in accidentally injured adults."

Patients with a history of affective disorders can have an exacerbation of these symptoms after a whiplash injury. Mayou et al[95] found that patients with a history of depression or anxiety were more likely to suffer from these states after their injuries. This, of course, does not mean that the symptoms are not real, but that there is the complicating factor of an underlying affective disorder that needs to be addressed as well.

For instance, Cicerone and Kalmar[202] found that there is no correlation between premorbid depression and depression after whiplash. They wrote, "The patients with a history of depression did not exhibit greater severity of self-reported post-concussive or emotional symptoms. It therefore appears unlikely that these patients' subjective complaints could be attributed solely to premorbid depression."

Litigation

There is still a great deal of controversy in regard to psychological symptoms and the role of litigation. Some physicians attribute emotional distress to chronic pain and the stress of litigation (or dealing with insurance companies); insurance companies claim that emotional symptoms are a sign of malingering. Where does the truth lie on this continuum?

Mayou et al[285] wrote, "It has often been alleged that the prospect of compensation is an important reason why many patients describe persistent symptoms and disability in the absence of abnormal physical findings. Our detailed information about the course and outcome of compensation proceedings is consistent with evidence in relation to neck symptoms from other prospective studies and shows that compensation is not a major determinant of any aspect of outcome."

Ratliff[320] wrote, "In a chapter of a new book, Evans[213] discusses the relation of litigation to symptoms, noting that many clinicians and certainly the insurance industry and the defense lawyers believe strongly in the concepts of secondary gain and compensation neurosis."

The notion of "accident neurosis," while still cited by some, has largely been laid to rest in the medical literature. Most of the current literature that claims that compensation is the primary motivation is not based upon carefully done study, but on anecdote alone.

Litigation, however, can have a dramatic negative effect on psychological well-being.[56] The very nature of litigation, with its confrontational structure, can result in stress. There can be anger at the insurance company for doubting the veracity of the patient's claim, fear that there will be no compensation, anxiety about impending court cases, or depression from feelings of helplessness.[74] The fact that litigation can take years to finalize is another complicating factor.

Treatment

The psychological symptoms of whiplash are one of the biggest problems for most physicians. Lehmann,[85] with unusual candor, wrote, "For orthopedic surgeons, dealing with the psychological aspect of injury is usually not an attractive part of the job. It does not lend itself to measurement or physical treatment. Its origins are outside the surgeons' area of interest and expertise..."

Medical treatment is moving more and more towards drug therapy for psychological symptoms. Of course, in some instances medications are appropriate, but it is important that the patient does not become dependent on these drugs and is aware of any potential side-effects. For more information about the drugs commonly used by whiplash patients, see the Medications section.

Emotional and social support need not be medically based. A study by Mynors-Wallis et al[104] reported that depressed patients improved more with problem solving therapy than with amitriptyline. Counselors, psychologists, or clergy can all be an excellent source of help. Just taking time to listen to a patient who has "been through the system" can be extremely therapeutic and give you important insights into the patient's condition.

The role of the physician

Some studies published in the last few years have elaborated on the role of the patient-doctor relationship as it relates to the psychological component of chronic pain. Patients seem to be keenly aware of physician expectations. Galer et al[221] found in their study that there was no relationship between the patient's expectations and results, but that there was a relationship between the *physician's* expectations and resulting pain relief.

"This suggests that physicians or health care providers who are asked to render therapies that are believed by the provider not to be efficacious may influence treatment outcomes in a negative way or, vice versa, if a provider strongly believes in a therapy, a positive outcome may be more likely."

Kouyanou et al[259] examined this problem, and explained specifically how physician behaviors can provoke certain patient reactions. The following chart illustrates these interactions.

Physician Behavior	Patient Responses
Over-investigating somatic or "organic" causes.	Adds to patient anxiety and uncertainty about the nature of their pain problems when (repeated) diagnostic tests fail to identify pathology.
Recommending measures not because of benefit, but because they feel pressured to help a desperate patient.	Fails to find a cure, and impedes on a patient's development of pain coping skills.
Misdirecting medication use; failing to provide specific instructions and advice.	Contributes to maintenance of disability among patients; medication should be given for a duration on a regular basis, not intermittently.
Directly or indirectly expressing skepticism if pain complaint is genuine.	Reinforces the patient's determination to maintain the sick role-to behave otherwise would confirm that it is "all in the mind." The patient feels stigmatized when physical pain is attributed to psychological causes.
Failing to offer adequate explanation for pain problems or an insufficient amount of background information.	Increases distress and anxiety levels. "Higher levels of information-giving, discussion of preventive care, and greater interview length contributed to patient satisfaction."
Clearly stating to the patient that appropriate investigation had been completed (and additional efforts would be fruitless).	Dissatisfied patients believed additional investigation would help, including their case histories and possible psychological problems or disorders.

Kouyanou,[258] in another study, further describes the negative effect a physician's attitude can have on patient recovery and response. "We observed that this group of patients reported a significantly higher frequency of direct disconfirmation of their pain by the doctors. We suggest that patients with medically unexplained symptoms are often exposed to attitudes that may paradoxically reinforce their determination to maintain the sick role, since to do otherwise would confirm the doctor's own view—that it was 'all in the mind' after all."

Post-Traumatic Stress Disorder

Post-Traumatic Stress Disorder (PTSD) is another controversial issue related to whiplash, and there is very little information about how often it occurs. It may be fairly common.[18] A study by Andersson et al[4] found that two years post-injury, 57% of whiplash patients were still suffering from "psychological distress." A number of other studies show that long-term psychological distress — even years after financial settlement — is fairly common after head injuries in general, and whiplash in particular. While the presence of psychological symptoms does not necessarily mean a diagnosis of PTSD, it is important for you to recognize this condition.

Symptoms

The following is the DSM-IV diagnostic criteria for Posttraumatic Stress Disorder:[27]

- Exposure to a traumatic event in which "the person experienced, witnessed, or was confronted with... actual or threatened death or serious injury, or a threat to the physical integrity of self or others." The patient must also have experienced the event with "intense fear, helplessness, or horror."
- "The traumatic event is persistently reexperienced" by distressing recollections of the event, distressing dreams, re-living of the event, or intense psychological or physical distress at exposure to cues that remind the patient of the trauma.
- Persistent avoidance of stimuli associated with the trauma or "numbing" of the senses. Examples are: avoiding thoughts of the event; avoiding activities, places, or people that arouse memories of the event; inability to recall important aspects of the trauma; diminished interest or participation in life activities; feelings of detachment; reduced range of emotional expression; or a lack of a sense of future.
- "Persistent symptoms of increased arousal." Examples are: insomnia, irritability, difficulty concentrating, or an exaggerated startle response.
- A duration of more than one month, with a disturbance in the person's social and work life.

Like all diagnostic criteria, the one for PTSD attempts to pigeon-hole human emotional reactions into narrow categories. Even if a person does not meet every criteria of PTSD, the presence of symptoms should be taken seriously.

Etiology

PTSD is not understood well by classical medicine. Cisler[19] wrote that the human body has "memory of injury," and this is true not only in the somatic sense, but in the psychological as well. In fact, with any chronic pain syndrome, it is critical to look at the whole person's situation for clues as to etiology and treatment.

The research shows a trend towards increased PTSD symptoms in patients with trauma to the head. Hickling et al[63] found that in a series of 20 accident victims with headache, 19 (or 95%) "had a diagnosable psychiatric disorder with 15 [or 75%] presenting with a post-traumatic stress disorder."

Bryant and Harvey[379] found that in a group of 79 patients who suffered mild traumatic brain injury as a result of a motor vehicle accident, 24% satisfied the criteria for PTSD six months after the accident.

Nielsen et al[376] suggests that the noise of a car crash may play some role in the stress associated with whiplash. One test subject who was a physician wrote this about his test experiences:

> "Although I was not injured or strained in any manner by these repeated rear-enders, the part that startled me the most was the drama of the noise. Rear-end crashes sound horrible, the whole vehicle reverberates with the echo of the impact. Yet upon looking at the bumpers afterwards, only minor dents were noted. It occurred to me that in persons who are emotionally fragile or dysfunctional, the fright from all this noise could be quite disturbing, and they might presume that certainly something could have happened to them. Fear can be very

convincing, and it is possible that for some individuals, this in itself could lead to the display of injury behaviour. This is a matter for further consideration."

Geisser et al[225] stated that their studies of PTSD and accident patients, "...suggest that PTSD symptoms in chronic pain patients are associated with increased pain and affective distress."

Buckley et al[190] wrote, "Thus, it may be that nagging physical injuries serve as a constant reminder of the trauma that helps to maintain, and in some cases exacerbate, participant's symptom presentations. Alternatively, it could be the case that trauma victims suffering from PTSD symptomatology are more sensitive to pain and thus give higher self-report ratings of pain and physical problems when questioned about the status of their injuries."

Amir et al[172] also reported that there seems to be a significant relationship between the amount of pain a patient reports and the presence of PTSD symptoms. This may be related to other studies that have found similarities between patients with fibromyalgia and PTSD.[234]

Shalev et al[380] found that there was a strong relationship between PTSD and depression following trauma, but that the two conditions were independent of each other.

There are a number of characteristics of the typical rear-end accident that increase the risk of PTSD symptoms.

1. The event is out of the victim's control. As stated in the DSM-IV, it involves "actual or threatened death, injury, or a threat to personal integrity." [27] In short, the person is "attacked" by the other automobile.

2. Also, in keeping with the DSM-IV, whiplash injuries involve feelings of helplessness and fear, especially when the person sees the accident coming, but can do nothing to prevent it.[27]

3. Many whiplash patients are phobic after their accidents — they're afraid to drive or to even ride in a car.[102,103,286]

4. The event is painful. Schreiber and Galai-Gat[131] wrote about an Israeli soldier who was hit in the face with a stone. The man was denied any pain medication for seven hours, until surgery was performed. He subsequently suffered from PTSD and chronic headaches. The authors wrote, "It is our experience that the core-trauma for the survivor may turn out to be an event or experience that took place before, or after, the event defined by others as catastrophic. [In this patient] the excruciating, prolonged and untreated pain he experienced while waiting for surgery overshadowed...the event of the injury..." They wrote that it was not the injury, but "the pain he experienced [that] was the traumatic element, the stressor that led to the development of PTSD." Of course, this man was in very severe pain, but it is not difficult to imagine the consequences of constant, serious whiplash pain that is not treated because the patient is believed to be "making it up."

5. The injury involves the head and neck. Radanov et al[120] found that headache "due to cervical pathology" was responsible for problems in attention and cognitive functioning. These symptoms are considered by many to be fictitiousness. Packard[166] found that when headache patients were asked what they wanted from their physicians, "an explanation of what was wrong," was the most common response. Packard et al[111] wrote, "One of the most frustrating experiences for patients may be to be told, 'Your MRI is normal; there is nothing wrong with you.' " Chronic head pain, combined with problems in memory or cognition can result in fear that permanent damage has been done, with concomitant depression or anxiety.

Treatment

Carlier et al[195] reported on the Self-Rating Scale for PTSD (SRS-PTSD)—a quick and efficient questionnaire that can be used to detect PTSD. The authors stress that this test does not replace the much more thorough interview required to diagnose PTSD.

Mayou et al[286] found that travel anxiety was a common symptom after motor vehicle accidents. "Travel anxiety after a motor vehicle accident is largely unrecognized in clinical practice and has been seen clinically as an occasional neurotic problem that might be associated with seeking compensation. Published literature is conflicting but the present study clearly shows that concern about travel is associated with considerable distress, behavioral change, and disability that is unrelated to the progress of compensation proceedings."

Much of the therapy for PTSD focuses on "desensitizing" the patient to the past trauma. Kuch et al,[80] in a group of car accident survivors, exposed the patients to things they were afraid of — driving, riding in a car, imagining their car accident. The researchers found that many of the patients were able to lessen their fears of driving in this manner.

Many of the patients you see with previously diagnosed PTSD will be taking medications. Kuch et al[80] had one third of their patients on diazepam (Valium) or lorazepam. Both of these drugs are in the benzodiazepine class, and are potentially addictive. (See Medications section for more information.) Hickling et al[63] reported on twenty cases of PTSD after motor vehicle accidents, and seventeen were on some kind of medication — analgesics, anti-headache, anti-depressants, or anti-anxiety. Fluoxetine (Prozac) is also commonly prescribed for PTSD patients.[150]

The Merck Manual[146] suggests psychotherapeutic treatment for PTSD, and has this to say about medications: "Antianxiety and antidepressant medications may be used adjunctively when necessary, but it should be remembered that this group of patients is particularly prone to develop drug dependency, so that prolonged pharmacotherapy generally is contraindicated."

Brown also found a high rate of substance abuse in PTSD patients.[13]

Geisser et al[225] wrote, "Behavioral treatment approaches such as cognitive-behavior therapy, systematic desensitization and relaxation training are often employed in the treatment of chronic pain and have also been efficacious in reducing symptoms of PTSD."

Since there is a strong pain component to PTSD, it seems prudent to work to relieve that. Massage therapy[41,43] and Therapeutic Touch[107] have been shown to relieve anxiety. Appropriate referral to a counselor for patients who are having psychological problems is recommended.

Chapter Five
Legal Issues

Malingering

"Two factors bedevil the field of whiplash. One is the belief that patients with neck pain after a motor vehicle accident are not suffering as a result of an organic lesion but have pain as a function of psychological disturbance. Therefore, some form of psychological assessment would appear to be mandatory, when evaluating patients with whiplash injury. The second factor is the fear that patients with whiplash may be malingering, because of the potential gain associated with insurance claims. For this reason, a diagnostic device which screened putative malingers would be attractive."[358]

As we've seen, whiplash can be physiologically very complex. The human body was not really designed to travel at highway speeds, and its structures are correspondingly fragile. Making matters more difficult, many of the symptoms of whiplash result from soft-tissue damage that is not revealed on radiological tests. Bogduk[11] wrote that the "seemingly bizarre features [of whiplash], which do not conform to some preconceived, classical neurological pattern, do not constitute evidence that the patient is somehow disturbed or not genuine." So, when we add the issues of liability and litigation, whiplash suddenly becomes even more complicated.

Although others had talked about "accident neurosis" as much as 100 years earlier, Miller[100] is still cited today in court cases. Miller described "accident neurosis" as such: "The general symptoms are remarkably constant, and amount to head pains (usually described as 'terrible,' 'terrific,' or 'agonizing'), exertional or postural dizziness, irritability, failure of concentration, and restlessness. Sleeplessness is volunteered in rather less than half, but in reply to leading questions the patient will usually claim insomnia of psychoneurotic pattern..." All of these allegedly "psychoneurotic " symptoms have been subsequently found to have organic origins. Miller claimed that virtually all patients recovered after settlement.

Miller is quoted as an expert by insurance companies. Interestingly, these statements by Miller were not from a controlled study, but from lectures he gave relating his anecdotal experience. Wallis et al[359] wrote, "The argument for compensation neurosis is based only on single cases or anecdotal evidence and is unsupported by any valid epidemiological or sociological studies. Indeed, formal studies and reviews have shown that financial compensation does not effect a cure and that despite settlement, a substantial proportion of patients suffers persistent pain and distress."

There is little scientific evidence that compensation neurosis is real.

Other studies are frequently used to show that the normal course of whiplash recovery is quick and uneventful immediately after legal settlement. The 1956 study by Gotten[52] is one of these studies. In the abstract of this study, it is stated, "After legal claims for damage were completed, 88% showed recovery, and over half of these had no residual complaints." In most articles disputing the reality of whiplash, authors use "88% recovered," without mentioning the fact that 34% still had symptoms after legal settlement.[40]

Gotten believed that whiplash was a fraudulent condition. He reported that "after the litigation, some patients divorced and remarried; others bought new homes, redecorated the home, and bought new cars. Such changes indicate the possibility that the illness had been used as a means of implementing psychological or other adjustments..." He also stated, "Many times the symptoms grew progessively worse over a period of weeks, although this was inconsistent with pathological possibilities."

Those patients whom Gotten admitted still had some symptoms were blamed for their symptoms: "Many who had some minor complaints of pain admitted upon questioning that they had not followed medical advice..."

It is an interesting fact that most of the literature that claims that whiplash is fictitious is either an editorial or selective review. Very, very few actual clinical trials find malingering to be a significant factor in recovery.

In an editorial, Pearce,[114] for instance, referred to just one study with his broad statement that "Alleged delayed onset is occasionally claimed but is not due to injury if there is an interval of more than 24 to 36 hours." The literature is full of evidence that this is not the case (see Delayed Onset). In this same editorial, Pearce also claims that "Migrainous features are not the result of whiplash injury," without making any literature references. The editorial concludes that "the evidence for consistent or relevant causal physical lesions remains flimsy."

More recently, Landy attempted to discredit the entire concept of chronic whiplash. The author showed little understanding of the basic biomechanics of collisions, the average age of his referenced studies was 21 years, and he claimed that injury was impossible without citing any engineering study since 1955!

The Lithuanian Study

In 1996, a study[336] appeared in *The Lancet* that received wide-spread media attention. This study set out to show that whiplash was not a real condition by surveying 202 Lithuanian drivers who had been involved in motor vehicle accidents.

The authors concluded that because few of the surveyed people reported chronic symptoms, long-term pain from whiplash was not a real issue.

The flaws in this study were numerous, and unfortunately, not reported by the mass media. Here is a summary of those flaws:

- The rate of whiplash has been calculated in western societies at 1 to 7 per 1,000 people.[340] This current study sent questionnaires to 240 accident subjects from a 3 year period in a city of 420,000 — a rate of .2 accidents per 1,000 people. This study does not make it clear whether all whiplash-type accident subjects were contacted, or whether they selectively picked them. If they picked all accidents that fit whiplash criteria, that would mean that rear-end accidents are far less common in Lithuania than they are here. This seems unlikely, as 17% of the control subjects had to be eliminated from the study because they had been in a previous accident.
- Of the 202 accident subjects, 157 (77.7%) were men, even though the medical literature has repeatedly shown that women are more likely to suffer long-term effects from whiplash.
- The researchers mailed out a total of 240 questionnaires, and 202 (84%) responded. The authors mention that they offered the participants entry into "a raffle for small prizes," but they don't mention what prizes these were. An 84% response rate seems very high for a survey sent out to the general public.
- The study states that it used Lithuania as the country of choice because of the nearly complete absence of automobile insurance and lack of knowledge of whiplash injuries. Possible confounding factors not addressed in this study include: the cultural attitudes of pain in Lithuania; the effects of poverty (in 1993, the legal minimum wage in Lithuania was just US$6.78 — *per month*[349]); the quality, make, and accident protective factors of the cars; the quality of police reports in a country where insurance coverage is rare; and the ability of patients to recall preexisting conditions up to 3 years after an injury.

Shortly after the publication of this study, professionals[267] from around the world added their criticisms:

One Norwegian professor dismissed the patient selection methods as invalid, and lack of use of safety belts (seatbelts have been found to *increase* the probability of whiplash injuries). He concluded that the Lithuanian study, "...is interesting as a research idea, but it should also be methodologically valid. The conclusions drawn from this study can hardly be justified by the data. They remain personal, unproven beliefs."

Two Dutch scientists also dismissed the selection methodology as flawed. They also questioned why there was no data on traffic density, number of accidents, and the severity of the injuries. They stated that the Lithuania study researchers, "...justify the selection of Lithuania as a study location by using the popular prejudice that the legal system has in fact created this disability. In our opinion, unsafe traffic is to blame, and sociocultural and legal circumstances encourage the submission of insurance claims..."

Finally, Dr. Michael Freeman and Dr. Arthur Croft wrote that, "Schrader and colleagues do not seem to have studied late-whiplash syndrome. They investigated 202 Lithuanian individuals who were involved in car accidents in which the police were summoned." They made the excellent point that the study should have studied people who had suffered a whiplash injury, not just people who had been in an accident. "When the accident exposed cohort was examined for those who had been exposed to acute whiplash, we found that only 15% (31 of 202) gave any indication of neck pain after their accident." Freeman and Croft then went on to reject all but two of the original group of patients as invalid. "As a result, none of Schrader's conclusions about this cohort relating to the natural progression of late whiplash are valid because of severe and fatal selection bias." [267]

The Opinion of Professionals on the Issue of Whiplash

There seems to be a strong bias in the medical community against patients with whiplash injuries. A survey[39] of physicians' attitudes on whiplash found that 31% of family practice doctors, 40% of neurosurgeons, and 46.8% of orthopedists believed that "prolonged whiplash symptoms [are] psychogenic in origin." The survey also found that 28% of family practice doctors, 52% of neurosurgeons, and 46% of orthopedists believed that "litigation factors [are] most responsible for whiplash symptoms."

The survey also elicited these comments from physicians:

A family practitioner: "I have a skeptical attitude on trauma where possible litigation may be at stake so my staff purposely channel away such patients."

A neurologist: "A large percentage of American health dollars are now spent in the unnecessary treatment of 'whiplash' and 'post-concussion syndrome.' "

A neurosurgeon: "Even though they have symptoms, the sooner they ignore them and get on with their lives the faster they will improve."

An orthopedist: "I strongly feel these injuries are seriously overtreated, overdiagnosed, over investigated and driven by litigation."

An orthopedist: "Legal system must address these fake syndromes."

The concept of accident neurosis is losing credibility as more information about the biomechanics of whiplash is being published. Mayou[287] wrote, "The terms accident or compensation neurosis were never completely accepted in psychiatry and are now demonstrably redundant. They should have no place in medical or legal discussion, but are still being used by doctors and lawyers."

These are the opinions. What are the facts? Is whiplash a "faked" condition?

Can Patients Fake Whiplash?

Wallis and Bogduk[358] studied this question by asking a group of 40 university students to fake a whiplash injury profile on the SCL-90-R—a symptom checklist that Wallis et al[359] had previously shown to be effective at objectively assessing the reality of whiplash pain.

The researchers found that the students "faking" whiplash had very high scores on all nine scales – much higher than the whiplash patients.

"Not only did students uniformly score higher, they scored highly across all subscales. It is in this latter respect that they differ from whiplash patients. Whiplash patients do not show randomly or uniformly elevated scores across subscales. They exhibit a characteristic profile with modest elevations on the somatisation, obsessive-compulsive, and depression subscales. The students were not able to reproduce this profile."

The authors conclude that, "it is very difficult for an ingenuine individual to fake a profile typical of a whiplash patient." [358]

Klimczak et al[254] similarly found that a group of subjects, even when informed about the nature of mild traumatic brain injury, could not convincingly fake it on a profile when asked.

In another study by Wallis et al[359] the authors wrote, "The argument for compensation neurosis is based only on single cases or anecdotal evidence and is unsupported by any valid epidemiological or sociological studies. Indeed, formal studies and reviews have shown that financial compensation does not effect a cure and that despite settlement, a substantial proportion of patients suffers persistent pain and distress."

Poor Diagnosis

Malingering can be used by insurance companies or physicians to shield their own ignorance. Patients who have a difficult diagnosis may simply be written off as malingering, when in fact the physician simply may not know enough to diagnose the problem. This assertion is backed up by an important study by Hendler et al,[241] who found that a large number of patients who had been "diagnosed" with psychogenic pain really had marked pathology that was not recognized by the treating physician. In fact, of these misdiagnosed patients, they found that upon careful examination, "98% of the patients had an organic origin for their pain complaints. In addition, 94.2% of the truly objective pain patients had demonstrated a marked physical abnormality responsible for their pain. It is evident from these figures, that without a thorough diagnostic evaluation, the label of psychogenic pain could be misapplied to an inadequately diagnosed patient, creating a self-fulfilling prophecy."

Litigation

Miller stated that patients were "cured by a verdict," and used the term compensation neurosis.[100]

MacNab[91] stated succinctly, "It is difficult to understand why patients should become neurotic if their head is thrown backwards and not if it is thrown forwards or from side to side, [and] if the symptoms...are purely the result of a litigation neurosis, it is difficult to explain why 45% of the patients should have their symptoms two years or more after settlement of their court action."

Balla[5] reported that in his group of accident victims, litigation did not cure the symptoms.

Gay and Abbott,[49] in one of the earliest studies of whiplash, stated, " In some patients, the aggravation of legal action was considered important, but, even after settlement, these patients were often partially disabled by recurrent nervous symptoms." As we have seen in the Post-Concussion section, these "nervous" symptoms could very easily been due to trauma, and not neurosis. Much of Gay and Abbott's confusion must be recognized as a lack of information, because at this time, the basic biomechanics of whiplash injury were still not understood.

In 1968, Schutt and Dohan[132] found that in a series of 74 women claiming whiplash injury, "the proportion (about 75%) of women with symptoms 6 to 26 months after the accident was as great in the groups not involved or no longer involved in litigation as in the group with pending litigation. In only one woman did litigation seem to be associated with prolonged subjective symptoms. She was the only one in whom muscle spasm was not detected one week after the accident."

A study by Galasko et al[46] reported that the rate of whiplash injuries in the UK has increased steadily from 1982 to 1991. "Our results suggest that the thought of litigation is not responsible for this increase."

Mendelson,[98] in his review of the literature, wrote, "Although it has been frequently claimed that the litigation process and the prospect of monetary compensation are the all-important factors in promoting continued disability in the absence of an obvious physical cause, there are also powerful psychological, cultural, and interpersonal factors operating, which have been all too frequently ignored in the evaluation and treatment of patients in compensable accidents." In regard to "accident neurosis," Mendelson wrote, "To the best of my knowledge, all studies published in the past 20 years have shown Miller's conclusions to be incorrect — indeed Kelly and Smith have termed them 'myths' — nevertheless, Miller remains the most frequently quoted authority on the prognosis of litigants after the settlement of their compensation claim." And, "...there is, at present, no justification for a medical practitioner to stand up in court and state that it is well known that litigants lose their symptoms and return to work shortly after their claim has been settled."

Any stressor can exacerbate a pain condition, and litigation is no exception. Greco et al[233] wrote, "Obviously, comparison of symptom presentation and treatment outcome among TMD patients with and without traumatic onset is complicated by the potential effects of compensation and litigation. Kolbinson and associates[375] reviewed the literature on postinjury temporomandibular disorders and concluded that these patients respond less well to treatment than did TMD patients whose symptoms were not attributed to specific traumatic events. These conclusions also held for litigating versus nonlitigating patients...In efforts to elucidate the effects of litigation status on post-traumatic TMD, Burgess and Dworkin[191] compared litigating and nonlitigating post-traumatic TMD patients. They found that the litigating group reported a greater number of pain sites initially, remained in treatment longer, and acknowledged a smaller percentage of improvement in symptoms following nonsurgical treatment modalities..." [233]

Swartzman et al[345] studied both patients who were currently involved in litigation and those who already settled. They wrote that "...chronic whiplash patients may be unique in the degree to which their pain is viewed with skepticism by both professionals and the general public. Accordingly, it may be particularly important to them that the extent of their pain is not underestimated. That is, whiplash patients may have a somewhat greater need than other chronic pain patients to communicate the extent of their pain. It should be noted that this is not the same as malingering. Our data do not suggest that chronic whiplash pain completely resolves and functionality is restored after litigation is concluded. Rather, it may be the case that these patients typically fear that pain will render them unable to work, or that their pain and associated disability will increase over time, leaving them with no recourse should they be unable to work in the future. They thus look to the litigation system to ensure some semblance of financial security." Another interesting finding was that the current litigants reported more pain immediately after the injury than did postlitigants. Although the study accounted for this statistically, it is possible that the current litigants had a more severe injury than did the postlitigants.

Mayou[287] wrote, "A recent report on behalf of the United Kingdom's Law Commission[264] interviewed a large number of recipients of awards from insurance companies and concluded that the amounts of settlement seemed to be modest in relation to injuries and losses, that they were often delayed, that they were spent appropriately, and indeed that there was strong evidence that losses, especially long-term losses, were underestimated."

In another study, Mayou[286] wrote, "The prolonged and frustrating pace of legal proceedings was the cause of very considerable anger and concern. This was especially so in those with more severe injuries (and therefore with the greatest need of compensation) whose cases generally took the longest time to resolve. Although there was no evidence that compensation was a major cause of longer term psychiatric and social problems, the prolonged and frustrating legal processes were a cause of stress and of financial difficulties and might reasonably be expected to have contributed to victims' overall views of satisfaction with outcome...Settlement did not seem to lead to any substantial change in social outcome, but it did result in subjects feeling a profound sense of relief and feeling able to move on from an unwanted preoccupation with the accident and its adverse effects on every day life and ambitions."

Norris and Watt[105] also found that litigation did not have an effect, but that the severity of symptoms determined who litigated and who did not.

Greenough and Fraser,[55] in a review of 300 work-related low back pain patients found that while compensation did tend to delay recovery, "settlement of the claim did not produce any improvement in the outcome," even after five years post-settlement.

The Lancet has been very skeptical of the reality of whiplash injuries. Nonetheless, *The Lancet* published an editorial[164] that stated, "Wickstrom et al leaves no doubt that complaints that were commonly regarded as neurotic — eg, blurring of vision and dizziness — have a firm organic basis, at least in the first few months and perhaps indefinitely."

Hoffman[66] stated, "What is clear is that many of these patients do suffer physically and emotionally and that their symptoms and disability continue long after their case is settled."

Chapter Six
Other Issues

Safety Devices and Whiplash Injuries

Head Restraints

If all modern passenger cars are required to have head restraints, and head restraints protect occupants from whiplash injuries, why do we still have so many whiplash cases? This issue has been studied extensively by a number of groups, and the answer is simple:

Head restraints are not designed to offer the best protection.

Each year, the Insurance Institute for Highway Safety reviews the protective ability of head restraints on hundreds of new vehicles. In 1995 and 1997, they found that fewer than 3% had the proper design to prevent injury.[339,363]

Even if a car does have an adequate head restraint, it doesn't mean that the driver knows how to use it. Viano and Gargan[353] documented the position of the head restraint in 1,915 cars that stopped at a city intersection. They found that only 10% of the occupants had the head restraint in the proper position to avoid hyperextension injuries. Only ¼ of the adjustable head restraints were in the "up" position. The authors estimate that if all of the adjustable head restraints had been in the up position, it would result in a 28% reduction of whiplash injury risk. The Insurance Institute for Highway Safety lowers the rating of vehicles with adjustable head restraints.[339]

We are likely to see some changes in this situation in the next few years. Researchers at SAAB have devised the "Saab Active Head Restraint" to protect occupants from whiplash.[364] In early tests with dummies, this restraint looks promising, although no studies have been published on the effectiveness on live subjects.

Volvo researchers are also working on the problem, and they are focusing on the entire seat/head restraint/shoulder belt structure itself to reduce the risk of injury.[274]

(For a more in-depth examination of the different issues related to head restraints, see our book *Low Velocity Whiplash Biomechanics*.)

> 90% of head restraints are adjusted improperly.

Neck and Chest Injuries From Seat Belts: A Mini-Review

The literature is quite clear that seat belts lower serious injuries and fatalities from high speed, frontal collisions. It is also clear that seat belts increase the risk of cervical soft-tissue injuries. In addition to the backward-forward movement of the head in a typical rear-end collision, seat belts add rotational forces to the head, making the injury more complex.[246] Bourbeau et al[186] found that in a survey of 3,927 accident victims, belted patients were 1.58 times more likely to suffer cervical strain than unbelted patients.

Thus, an awareness of the different types of injuries seat belts can cause is critical. The following are some of the documented effects of seat belt injuries.

Breast Injuries

Breast injuries from seat belts have been documented in the medical literature since 1972. A more recent study[206] reported on breast injuries from seat belts in five women who were examined with mammography and sonography. The exams found cysts or bands of increased density in all five women, indicative of contusions, lipid cysts, and calcifications of the breast tissue. "With the increased use of seatbelts with shoulder restraints, injury of the breast of sufficient severity results in fat necrosis...On occasion, as for one of the patients described in this report, the particles may have a more suspicious appearance and warrant biopsy."

Heart and Sternal Injuries

This is another type of injury well-documented. Restifo and Kelen[323] report on a case of sternal fracture from a seatbelt injury, in which the only symptoms were sternal pain. Another study found that seat belt damage to the chest can be more invasive: "Both seatbelt-related and major trunkal injuries have a relatively high (25-30%) incidence of some degree of pericardial or myocardial trauma, evidenced by a definite pericardial effusion on echocardiography."[189] None of these patients had serious consequences from the sternal injuries, but long-term pain was not studied.

Thyroid Injury

One report[265] related the case of a 64-year-old man "with no prior history of thyroid disease [who] presented with 2 months of worsening pain in the left side of his neck. He recently had purchased a used car and noticed the seat belt was too tight, tending to rub the left side of his neck. On physical examination, the left lobe of the thyroid gland was moderately enlarged and tender; the right lobe was normal." Radiological tests found traumatic thyroiditis. One month after replacing the seat belt, the patient was asymptomatic. The authors recommend watching for thyroid trauma from seat belt injuries.

Another report discussed rupture of the thyroid gland by blunt trauma to the neck.[330]

Laryngeal Trauma

The possibility of damage to the thyroid gland is elucidated further from studies that have found laryngeal fracture and trauma from seat belt injuries. One study reported on fracture of the larynx after an auto accident although the study does not mention seat belt involvement.[343]

A second article[235] reports on laryngeal trauma from a auto injury, in which a 26-year-old woman was rear-ended. The woman reported to the hospital with "moderate tenderness over the left thyroid cartilage ala." Two hours later she began to cough blood and became hoarse. She required surgery for laryngeal laceration. "The mechanism of injury may have been anterior movement of the upper body with leftward twisting of the head and neck because of the shoulder belt crossing the left side of the neck. This would result in left-to-right lateral compression and rotation of the larynx, which would account for the injury." The symptoms of laryngeal trauma include hoarseness; difficulty or pain when swallowing; trouble with speaking; difficulty breathing; or pain. Hartmann et al found that symptoms may take as long as 48 hours to present.[239]

Carotid Artery Injury

A recent study[204] looked at Internal Carotid Artery (ICA) injuries after trauma. The researchers studied 60 patients with dissection of the ICA. Ten of these had injuries from trauma, and these included traffic accidents. Thirty six of the cases were determined to be "spontaneous disections," with no known etiology, but the authors write:

"The term 'spontaneous dissection' implies that there has been no trauma causing the pathology. According to some authors, the role of trivial trauma cannot be excluded (Hart et al[238]). In such cases, the proposed mechanism is an hyperextension or a lateral flexion of the neck which stretches the ICA over the transverse processes of the upper cervical vertebrae (Anson et al[175])." [204]

Two new studies relate cases of non-direct trauma to the neck as cause of ICA dissection.

The first study[248] was the case of a woman in a head-on collision who suffered a severe whiplash injury, and who also was found to have bilateral ICA damage. Symptoms of ICA dissection were not recognized for the first few days. The authors discuss the mechanism of injury: "Carotid artery dissection has been reported to result from hyperextension of the neck causing longitudinal traction over the carotid arteries with their impingement against the lateral mass of the atlas and transverse processes of the spine. It has also been reported following acute hyperflexion injury, causing compression of the vessel between mandible and spine. Besides these, other contributing factors reported in the literature are injury caused by a high riding shoulder strap of a safety belt, a long styloid process, mandible fracture, and traction of the hypoglossal nerve against the carotid artery. The above described mechanisms of hyperextension and hyperflexion injuries are usually associated with rotatory force and therefore are more likely to cause unilateral carotid arterial dissection because this maneuver will provide tension on one side while relaxing the vessel on the opposite side." They warn that such lesions may not appear immediately, and that "This delay may vary from a few hours to as long as 14 years but the usual delay is 3 hours to several days after injury." [248]

The second study[266] was a case of 50-year-old man who also did not have direct trauma to the neck, but was found to have dissection of the ICA two weeks after a car accident. In this man's case, dissection of the ICA resulted in dysfunction of the hypoglossal nerve. This dysfunction presented in the form of disturbed speech, difficulty swallowing, and problems moving his tongue.

Other studies that have documented the the role of seat belts in ICA injury are those by Reddy et al,[321] Benito et al,[177] and Chedid et al.[197]

The symptoms of ICA trauma can range from hematoma, to hemicrania, Horner's syndrome, paralysis, unilateral facial weakness, hemianesthesia, and aphasia." [196]

Airbag Injuries

Airbags were developed to save lives, and in serious head-on collisions they do so. Unfortunately, airbags also can cause injury themselves. That injuries can be caused by airbags becomes obvious when one considers the force with which airbags open. "The velocity of deployment has been measured by the National Highway Traffic Safety Administration (NHTSA) and *averages 144 mph with maximum velocities of 211 mph reported.*" [338] [emphasis added] These velocities are of the airbag itself, irrespective of the severity of the collision. "When airbags for passenger vehicles were still in the research and development phase, the automotive industry conducted tests that clearly demonstrated the potential for fatal injuries associated with airbag deployment. The industry itself came to the conclusion that the life-saving airbag could also be life-threatening." [338]

The following types of injuries have been documented in the literature:

- Injuries from the airbag module cover. One study[338] reported avulsion of the thumb after a patient braced herself against the airbag cover. Another woman in a 5 mph accident, with minor damage to the car, "sustained multiple fractures of the right upper extremity which included a severely comminuted fracture of the ulnar olecranon and ulnar shaft, a radial head dislocation, a comminuted fracture of the medial epicondyle with elbow dislocation of the humeral shaft." A third woman died from severe head injuries from an airbag after her car grazed a guardrail; the car sustained minimal damage, and five other passengers in the car had either no or very slight injuries.[338] Those at the greatest risk for such injuries are those drivers who are shorter and sit closer to the steering wheel.[296]
- Injuries from the force of the airbag itself. These include eye injuries,[332] broken arms, and facial injuries. Airbags can either directly impact a body part, resulting in trauma, or the upper extremity can be thrown from the force of the trauma into the face or a hard surface of the vehicle. One case in particular sums up the kinds of injuries that can result from even minor collisions: "A 1989 Dodge Daytona struck the front of an oncoming vehicle that had crossed the center line. Left front corner impact damage to the Daytona was very minor. The 29-year-old female driver (height, 170 cm; mass 65 kg) was wearing her lap-shoulder belt and had her seat at mid position. The driver's left hand was propelled into the windshield by airbag deployment as indicated by the star burst pattern on the windshield. The driver's injuries included a bruise of the left hand, from the windshield impact, a cervical spine strain, and bruises of the chest and right hip from the belt restraint webbing."[244] All this, in an accident with "very minor" damage.
- Another patient, also in an accident with minor car damage, also suffered serious injuries. In this case, the 59-year-old man experienced fracture of the right ulna and radius, and the force of his arm hitting his face fractured his nose and the anterior wall of the right maxillary sinus, and chipped two teeth.[244]
- Other studies have suggested a link between airbag deployment and TMJ injury and pain.[211,233]

Anti-Lock Brakes

Evans and Gerrish[212] studied police records from 1992 and 1993 for five states, looking specifically at rear end collsions. The authors found that cars with anti-lock brakes (ABS) are significantly less likely to rear-end another car. However, cars with ABS are 30% more likely to be rear-ended themselves.

Children and Whiplash

Very little literature has been published on the issue of children and whiplash. Only recently have crash tests used dummies in a child's size, and no experimental tests have been done on rear end collisions with children.

Over the years, we have heard numerous reports from readers that insurance companies routinely claim that children cannot be injured in rear end collisions. The existing literature, however, disputes these claims.

Lynch et al[275] reported on a case of a 6-year-old girl who became quadriplegic when the car she was riding in was rear ended at 35 mph by a truck.

Physicians at The Children's Hospital of Alabama stressed the importance of addressing cervical spine injuries in children.[230]

First, they discuss the anatomy of the pediatric spine. "Previous studies of cervical spine injury in pediatric patients characterize it as 'fundamentally different from its adult counterpart.' Although due in part to differences in mechanism of injury between adults and children, a large degree of the variance is attributed to anatomic differences in the developing pediatric cervical spine. These features and their assumed effects include the disproportionately large mass of the head and relatively underdeveloped neck musculature of the infant and young child that create a bending moment at impact that is very large relative to the neck muscle strength; wedge-shaped vertebral bodies facilitating anterior articulating facets that predispose the child's cervical spine to greater mobility than that seen in adults, particularly in the upper three to four cervical spine segments; and the relative elasticity and laxity of the interspinous ligaments, posterior joint capsules, and cartilaginous end plates in the pediatric patient. While most of the neural arches close and the dens synchondrosis fuses by approximately 3 years of age, a child's cervical spine does not fully take on the characteristics of the adult spine until he or she approaches 8 years of age. By this time the anterior wedging of the vertebral bodies disappears, the articulating facets become more vertically oriented, and the tensile strength of the ligaments and capsules increases.

"These anatomic properties are believed to have several important implications. The ligamentous laxity of the young pediatric spine serves to absorb and distribute traumatic forces, protecting against injury to the osseous elements and, more importantly, the spinal cord. Since most pediatric injuries are of a low-energy nature, cervical spine involvement is much less common in acutely injured children than in adults. With higher energy forces, such as are applied with rapid deceleration or hyperflexion-extension mechanisms, lethal distraction or shear forces with significant cord ischemia or infarction may occur, even in the absence of osseous fracture or subluxation."

The authors found that few cervical spine injuries were found in children who were properly restrained in automobiles. They do raise an important concern regarding these types of injuries, however. "Two of the remaining children…ages 5 and 6 years, respectively, were restrained in lap-shoulder belts and sustained isolated cervical spine injuries in motor vehicle crashes. Although this may be considered 'age-appropriate' restraint given current laws and practices in the United States, questions have been raised whether appropriate restraint mechanisms for young school-aged children in fact exist. Several authors have pointed out that lap-shoulder belts not only provide 'no protection' for the cervical spine but may actually be the cause of certain types of injuries, including cervical spine fractures, particularly in the 4- to 9-year age group.[170,302,334] Because they are designed for the adult body configuration, they fail to account for the fact that, because the child's sitting height is less than that of the average adult, the child's center of gravity is often located on the torso above the level of the lap belt. The greater proportion of body mass above the belt may cause greater forward motion and a greater chance for head impact. The shoulder portion of the belt may ride over the young child's face and neck."

This information may be of value to physicians working with children accident victims, as insurance companies will sometimes claim that children do not suffer injuries from whiplash.

Psychological problems after motor vehicle accidents have also been documented in children. Di Gallo et al[205] studied PTSD in children after car crashes, and reported, "Accidents, although often frightening and distressing for victims, were mostly considered minor, after the initial shock, by parents, friends, and relatives. Subjects were often told they had been fortunate and their condition could have been worse. Little opportunity was left to discuss feelings, such as fears or helplessness, and enforced normality was imposed upon several victims...Parents were commonly unaware of their avoiding behaviour, but acknowledged tension, mood swings and tantrums in their child, leading to frequent arguments."

The children most likely to develop symptoms of PTSD were those who were younger (those who could not understand what had happened to them) and those who were very distressed at the time of the accident. The authors stress that these children should be followed very closely, that the families should be made aware of possible reactions and symptoms, and that referral to a mental health professional may be warranted in certain cases.

Medications

Many people are prescribed medications after whiplash injuries, and it is important for you to know what the most common drugs are so that you can recognize any potential adverse effects. The following is a listing of the different categories of drugs used, the common trade names, their indications, and things to look for.

Benzodiazepines

Common types: Diazepam (Valium), Alprazolam (Xanax), Lorazepam (Ativan).

General characteristics: Centrally-acting sedative, hypnotic, and anti-anxiety drugs.

Uses: Anxiety and tension, muscle spasms, sleep disturbances, myofascial pain.

Concerns: "All antianxiety agents have the ability to cause psychological and physical dependence. Withdrawal symptoms usually start within 12-48 hr after stopping the drug and last for 12-48 hr...Abrupt withdrawal may be accompanied by coma, convulsions, and even death."

Adverse Effects: Drowsiness, lightheadedness, fatigue and tiredness, impaired coordination, constipation, skin rashs, dry mouth, dizziness, increased appetite, sexual dysfunction.[88]

Muscle Relaxants

Common types: Carisoprodol (Soma), Chlorzoxazone (Paraflex), Cyclobenzaprine (Flexeril), Metaxalone (Skelaxin), Methocarbamol (Delaxin)

General Characteristics: Muscle relaxants work via the central nervous system, decreasing muscle tone and involuntary movement throughout the body. They also have some analgesic properties.

Uses: Muscle spasm, tension headaches, inflammation.

Concerns: Should not be used with MAOI or tricyclic anti-depressants, as severe symptoms can result. Dosage must be tapered when discontinuing treatment to prevent withdrawal symptoms.

Adverse Effects: Dry mouth, drowsiness, weakness, paresthesia, insomnia, dizziness, tachycardia, blurred vision, urinary retention.[88]

Non-Steroidal Anti-Inflammatory Drugs (NSAIDs)

Common types: Acetylsalicylic acid (aspirin), Ibuprofen, Indomethacin (Indocin), Naproxen (Naprosyn).

General Characteristics: Decrease levels of prostoglandins, thereby reducing inflammation. Also have analgesic properties.

Uses: Inflammation, pain, arthritis.

Concerns: Should not be used by pregnant or lactating women. Overuse of this class of drugs can lead to gastrointestinal damage.

Adverse Effects: Ulcer, heartburn, nausea, vomiting, dyspepsia, indigestion, abdominal cramps, dizziness, drowsiness, vertigo, headaches, nervousness, anxiety.[88]

Narcotic Analgesics

Common types: Codeine, Fiorinal, Meperidine (Demerol), Percocet, Percodan, Propoxyphene (Darvon).

General Characteristics: These drugs affect the central nervous system, decreasing pain.

Uses: Moderate or severe acute pain. Fiorinal is used for tension headaches. Many whiplash patients are prescribed these drugs for myofascial pain.

Concerns: All of these drugs are potentially addictive. They should not be used for long-term treatment of pain. Also, caution should be used if using alcohol, antianxiety drugs, antidepressants, or muscle relaxants, as these can cause potentially serious additive adverse effects.

Adverse Effects: Respiratory depression, apnea, dizziness, lightheadedness, sedation, lethargy, headache, nausea, vomiting, constipation, skin rashes, urinary retention.[88]

Selective Serotonin Reuptake Inhibitors (SSRIs)

Common types: Fluoxetine Hydrochloride (Prozac), Paroxetine Hydrochloride (Paxil), Sertraline Hydrochloride (Zoloft).

General Characteristics: Drug prevents reuptake of serotonin in the body, increasing serotonin levels.

Uses: Indicated for depression, commonly used for depression resulting from chronic pain.

Concerns: These drugs have a large number of side-effects, and are prescribed very often. These drugs can also cause headache and muscle pain, complicating the treatment of whiplash injuries.

Adverse Effects: Headache, insomnia, anxiety, nervousness, dizziness, fatigue, sedation, sexual dysfunction, decreased concentration, agitation, abnormal dreams, paranoid reactions, suicidal ideations, and blurred vision. (This is just a short, general list of symptoms. For each specific drug, there are dozens more documented adverse effects.)[88]

Tricyclic Antidepressants

Common Types: Amitriptyline (Elavil), Desipramine (Norpramin), Imipramine (Tofranil), Nortriptyline (Pamelor).

General Characteristics: Prevent the reuptake of norepinephrine or serotonin, or both. They all have a strong sedative effect.

Uses: Depression, chronic pain.

Concerns: Should not be used with any other antidepressants or alcohol. Should not be used during pregnancy or lactation.

Adverse Effects: Confusion, anxiety, restlessness, insomnia, nightmares, hallucinations, delusions, mania, headache, dizziness, difficulty concentrating, panic reactions, fatigue, blurred vision, nausea, vomiting, fainting, and urinary retention.[88]

Warning

Limitations of space prevent a thorough listing of all adverse effects of these drugs. If a patient or client of yours is presenting with what you suspect to be an adverse reaction, please check the *Physician's Desk Reference*, and have the patient check with his or her pharmacist or doctor.

Some of these drugs may cause severe withdrawal symptoms, and should not be discontinued without medical supervision.[88] A referral to another medical provider may be required.

Appendix

The Neck Pain Disability Index

The Neck Pain Disability Index is a questionnaire developed by Dr. Howard Vernon, DC, designed to assess whiplash patients.[389] The survey is a modification of the Oswestry Low Back Disability Index. Each category contains 6 possible answers, scored from 0 to 5. Scores are totaled, and a rating is determined: 0-4 = No disability; 5-14 = Mild disability; 15-24 = Moderate disability; 25-34 = Severe Disability; 35-50 = Complete disability. The test has been studied a number of times and has been found to be a reliable and accurate assessment of neck pain disability. On the following page is a copy of the survey, and as the article states, "its duplication and use is encouraged."

This survey provides a simple tool for quantifying neck pain disability, and the author suggests using it to evaluate a patient's progress and to determine severity of disability. Please feel free to copy the following page and use this survey in your practice.

This questionnaire has been designed to give the doctor information as to how your neck pain has affected your ability to manage in everyday life. Please answer every section and mark in each section only the ONE box which applies to you. We realize you may consider that two of the statements in any one section relate to you, but just mark the **one** box that most clearly describes your problem.

Section 1 – Pain Intensity
❑ I have no pain at the moment.
❑ The pain is very mild at the moment.
❑ The pain is moderate at the moment.
❑ The pain is fairly severe at the moment.
❑ The pain is the worst imaginable at the moment.

Section 2 – Personal Care
❑ I can look after myself normally without causing extra pain.
❑ I can look after myself normally but it causes extra pain.
❑ It is painful to look after myself and I am slow and careful.
❑ I need some help but manage most of my personal care.
❑ I need help every day in most aspects of self care.
❑ I do not get dressed, I wash with difficulty and stay in bed.

Section 3 – Lifting
❑ I can lift heavy weights without extra pain.
❑ I can lift heavy weights but it gives me extra pain.
❑ Pain prevents me from lifting heavy weights off the floor, but I can manage if they are conveniently positioned, for example on a table.
❑ I can lift very light weights.
❑ I cannot lift or carry anything at all.

Section 4 – Reading
❑ I can read as much as I want to with no pain in my neck.
❑ I can read as much as I want to with slight pain in my neck.
❑ I can read as much as I want with moderate pain in my neck.
❑ I can't read as much as I want because of moderate pain in my neck.
❑ I can hardly read at all because of severe pain in my neck.
❑ I cannot read at all.

Section 5 – Headaches
❑ I have no headaches at all.
❑ I have slight headaches which come infrequently.
❑ I have moderate headaches which come infrequently.
❑ I have moderate headaches which come frequently.
❑ I have severe headaches which come frequently.
❑ I have headaches almost all the time.

Section 6 – Concentration
❑ I can concentrate fully when I want to with no difficulty.
❑ I can concentrate fully when I want to with slight difficulty.
❑ I have a fair degree of difficulty in concentrating when I want to.
❑ I have a lot of difficulty in concentrating when I want to.
❑ I have a great deal of difficulty in concentrating when I want to.
❑ I cannot concentrate at all.

Section 7 – Work
❑ I can do as much work as I want to.
❑ I can only do my usual work, but no more.
❑ I can do most of my usual work, but no more.
❑ I cannot do my usual work.
❑ I can hardly do any work at all.
❑ I can't do any work at all.

Section 8 – Driving
❑ I can drive my car without any neck pain.
❑ I can drive my car as long as I want with slight pain in my neck. I can drive my car as long as I want with moderate pain in my neck.
❑ I can't drive my car as long as I want because of moderate pain in my neck.
❑ I can hardly drive at all because of severe pain in my neck.
❑ I can't drive my car at all.

Section 9 – Sleeping
❑ I have no trouble sleeping.
❑ My sleep is slightly disturbed (less than 1 hour sleepless).
❑ My sleep is mildly disturbed (1-2 hours sleepless).
❑ My sleep is moderately disturbed (2-3 hours sleepless).
❑ My sleep is greatly disturbed (3-5 hours sleepless).
❑ My sleep is completely disturbed (5-7 hours sleepless).

Section 10 – Recreation
❑ I am able to engage in all my recreation activities with no neck pain at all.
❑ I am able to engage in all my recreation activities, with some pain in my neck.
❑ I am able to engage in most, but not all, of my usual recreation activities because of pain in my neck.
❑ I am able to engage in a few of my usual recreation activities because of pain in my neck.
❑ I can't do any recreation activities at all.

Bibliography

1.   Algers G, Pettersson K, Hildingsson C, Toolanen G. Surgery for chronic symptoms after whiplash injury: follow-up of 20 cases. Acta Orthopedia Scandinavica 1993;64:654-656.

2.   Allen ME, Weir-Jones I, Motiuk DR et al. Acceleration perturbations of daily living: a comparison to whiplash. Spine 1994;19:1285-1290.

3.   Allen MJ, Barnes MR, Bodiwala GG. The effect of seat belt legislation on injuries sustained by car occupants. Injury: The British Journal of Accident Surgery 1985;16;471-476.

4.   Andersson AL, Dahlback LO, Allebeck P. Psychosocial consequences of traffic accidents: a two year follow-up. Scandinavian Journal of Social Medicine 1994;22:299-302.

5.   Balla JI, Moraitis S. Knights in armour: a follow-up study of injuries after legal settlement. Medical Journal of Australia 1970;1:355-361.

6.   Balla J, Karnaghan J. Whiplash headache. Clinical and Experimental Neurology 1987;23:179-182.

7.   Barnsley L, Lord SM, Wallis BJ, Bogduk N. The prevalence of chronic cervical zygapophysial joint pain after whiplash. Spine 1995;20:20-25.

8.   Beneliyahu DJ. Chiropractic management and manipulative therapy for MRI documented cervical disk herniation. Journal of Manipulative and Physiological Therapeutics 1994;17:177-185.

9.   Blau JN, MacGregor EA. Migraine and the neck. Headache 1994;34:88-90.

10. Boden SD et al. Abnormal resonance scans of the lumbar spine in asymptomatic subjects. Journal of Bone and Joint Surgery 1990;72-A:403-408.

11. Bogduk N. Post whiplash syndrome. Australian Family Physician 1994;23:2303-2307.

12. Boline PD, Kassak K, Bronfort G, Nelson C, Anderson AV. Spinal manipulation vs. amitriptyline for the treatment of chronic tension-type headaches: a randomized clinical trial. Journal of Manipulative and Physiological Therapeutics 1995;18;3:148-154.

13. Brown PJ, Recupero PR, Stout R. PTSD substance abuse comorbidity and treatment utilization. Addictive Behavior 1995;20:251-254.

14. Burke JP, Orton HP, West J et al. Whiplash and its effect on the visual system. Graefe's Arch Clinical and Experimental Opthalmology 1992;230:335-339.

15. Capistrant TD. Thoracic outlet syndrome in whiplash injury. Annals of Surgery 1977;185:175-178.

16. Carette S. Whiplash injury and chronic neck pain. New England Journal of Medicine 1994;330:1083-4.

17. Chemtob CM, Hamada RS, Roitblat HL, Muraoka MY. Anger, impulsivity, and anger control in combat-related posttraumatic stress disorder. Journal of Consulting and Clinical Psychology 1994;62:827-832.

18. Chibnall JT, Duckro PN. Post-traumatic stress disorder in chronic post-traumatic headache patients. Headache 1994;34:357-361.

19. Cisler TA. Whiplash as a total-body injury. Journal of the American Osteopathic Association 1994;94:145-148.

20. Cotton P. Symptoms may return after carpal tunnel surgery. Journal of the American Medical Association 1991;265;15;1922-1925.

21. Croft AC, Foreman SM. *Whiplash Injuries: The Cervical Acceleration Deceleration Syndrome.* Baltimore, Williams & Wilkins, 1988.

22. Croft P, Schollum J, Silman A. Population study of tender point counts and pain as evidence of fibromyalgia. BMJ 1994;309:696-9.

23. Cyriax J. Rheumatic headache. The British Medical Journal 1938;2:1367-1368.

24. Davis SJ, Teresi LM, Bradley WG, Ziemba MA, Bloze AE. Cervical spine hyperextension injuries: MR findings. Radiology 1991;180:245-251.

25. de Jong PTVM, de Jong JMBV, Cohen B, et al. Ataxia and nystagmus induced by injection of local anesthetics in the neck. Annals of Neurology 1977;1:240-246.

26. Deans GT, Magalliard JN, Kerr M, Rutherford WH. Neck sprain — a major cause of disability following car accidents. Injury 1987;18:10-12.

27. *Diagnostic and Statistical Manual of Mental Disorders* (4th Edition), American Psychiatric Association, 1994.

28. Dorman TA. Letter. The Lancet 1991;338:1208.

29. Duckro PN, Chibnall JT, Tomazic TJ. Anger, depression, and disability: a path analysis of relationships in a sample of chronic posttraumatic headache patients. Headache 1995;35:7-9.

30. Duckro PN, Schultz KT, Chibnall JT. Migraine as a sequela to chronic low back pain. Headache 1994;34:279-281.

31. Duckro PN, Chibnall JT, Greenberg MS. Myofascial involvement in chronic post-traumatic headache. Headache Quarterly 1995;6:34-38.

32. Duckro PN, Schultz KT, Chibnall JT. Migraine as a sequela to chronic low back pain. Headache 1994;34:279-281.

33. Dvorak J, Hayek J, Zehnder R. CT-functional diagnostics of the rotatory instability of the upper cervical spine. Part 2. An evaluation of healthy adults and patients with suspected instability. Spine 1987;12:726-731.

34. Dvorak J, Gauchat MH, Valach L. The outcome of surgery for lumbar disc herniation. 1. A 4-17 years' follow-up with emphasis on somatic aspects. Spine 1988;13:1418-22.

35. Ellison DW, Wood VE. Trauma-related thoracic outlet syndrome. Journal of Hand Surgery 1994;19B:424-426.

36. Ettlin TM, Kischka U, Reichmann S, Radii EW et al. Cerebral symptoms after whiplash injury of the neck: a prospective clinical and neuropsychological study of whiplash injury. Journal of Neurology, Neurosurgery, and Psychiatry 1992;55:943-948.

37. Evans RW. Some observations on whiplash injuries. The Neurology of Trauma 1992;10;4;975-997.

38. Evans RW. The postconcussion syndrome and the sequelae of mild head injury. Neurology of Trauma 1992;10:815-847.

39. Evans RW, Evans RI, Sharp MJ. The physician survey on the post concussion and whiplash syndromes. Headache 1994;34:268-274.

40. Farbman AA. Neck sprain: associated factors. Journal of the American Medical Association 1973 223:1010-1015.

41. Field T, Morrow C, Valdeon C et al. Massage reduces anxiety in child and adolescent psychiatry patients. Journal of the American Acadamy of Child and Adolescent Psychiatry 1992;31:125-131.

42. Frankel VH. Temporomandibular joint pain syndrome following deceleration injury to the cervical spine. Bulletin of Hospital Joint Dis 1969;26:47-51.

43. Fraser J, Kerr JR. Psychophysiological effects of back massage on elderly institutionalized patients. Journal of Advanced Nursing 1993;18:238-245.

44. Friedman D, Flanders A, Thomas C, Millar W. Vertebral artery injury after acute cervical spine trama: rate of occurrence as detected by MR angiography and assessment of clinical consequences. American Journal of Radiology 1995;164;443-447.

45. Friedmann LW, Marin EL, Padula PA. Biomechanics of cervical trauma, in *Painful Cervical Trauma: Diagnosis and Rehabilitative Treatment of Neuromuscular Injuries*, Ed. Tollison CD, Satterthwaite JR 1992;10-19.

46. Galasko CSB, Murray PM, Pitcher M et al. Neck sprains after road traffic accidents: a modern epidemic. Injury 1993;24:155-157.

47. Gargan MF, Bannister GC. The rate of recovery following whiplash injury. European Spine Journal 1994;3:162-4.

48. Gargan MF, Bannister GC. Long-term prognosis of soft-tissue injuries of the neck. Journal of Bone and Joint Surgery 1990;72B:901-3.

49. Gay JR, Abbott KH. Common whiplash injuries of the neck. Journal of the American Medical Association 1953;152:1698-1704.

50. Gebhard JS, Donaldson DH, Brown CW. Soft-tissue injuries of the cervical spine. Orthopedic Review 1994:9-17.

51. Gobel H, Hamouz V, Hansen C, et al. Chronic tension-type headache: amitriptyline reduces clinical headache-duration and experimental pain sensitivity but does not alter pericranial muscle activity 93 readings. Pain 1994;59:241-249.

52. Gotten N. Survey of one hundred cases of whiplash injury after settlement of litigation. Journal of the American Medical Association 1956;162:865-867.

53. Grable HR. Abnormal findings on magnetic resonance imaging in a group of motor vehicle accident patients with low back pain. American Journal of Medical Quality 1993;Winter:194-196.

54. Graff-Radford SB, Jaeger B, Reeves JL. Myofascial pain may present clinically as occipital neuraglia. Neurosurgery 1986;19;4:610-613.

55. Greenough CG, Fraser RD. The effects of compensation on recovery from low back injury. Spine 1989;14:947-955.

56. Guest GH, Drummond PD. Effect of compensation on emotional state and disability in chronic back pain. Pain 1992;48:125-130.

57. Ham LP, Andrasik F, Packard RC, Bundrick CM. Psychopathology in individuals with post-traumatic headaches and other pain types. Cephalgia 1994;14:118-126.

58. Hamer AJ, Gargan MF, Bannister GC, Nelson RJ. Whiplash injury and surgically treated cervical disc disease. Injury 1993;24:549-550.

59. Haslett RS, Duvall-Young J, McGalliard JN. Traumatic retinal angiopathy and seat belts: pathogenesis of whiplash injury. Eye 1994;8:615-617.

60. Hatch JP, Schoenfeld LS, Boutros NN, Seleshi E, Moore PJ, Cyr-Provost M. Anger and hostility in tension-type headache. Headache 1991;31:302-304.

61. Heise AP, Laskin DM, Gervin AS. Incidence of temporomandibular joint symptoms following whiplash injury. Journal of Oral and Maxillofacial Surgery 1992;50:825-828.

62. Hendler NH, Kozikowski JG. Overlooked physical diagnoses in chronic pain patients involved in litigation. Psychosomatics 1993;34:494-501.

63. Hickling EJ, Blanchard EB, Silverman DJ, Schwarz SP. Motor vehicle accidents, headaches and post-traumatic stress disorder: assessment findings in a consecutive series. Headache 1992;32:147-151.

64. Hildingsson C, Toolanen G. Outcome after soft-tissue injury of the cervical spine. Acta Orthopedic Scandinavica 1990;61:357-359.

65. Hodgson SP, Grundy M. Whiplash injuries: their long-term prognosis and its relationship to compensation. Neuro-Orthopedics 1989;7:88-91.

66. Hoffman BF. The demographic and psychiatric characteristics of 110 personal injury litigants. Bulletin of the American Academy of Psychiatry and Law 1991;19:227-236.

67. Hohl M. Soft-tissue injuries of the neck in automobile accidents: factors influencing prognosis. Journal of Bone Joint Surgery 1974;56A:1675-1682.

68. Hong CZ, Simons DG. Response to treatment for pectoralis minor myofascial pain syndrome after whiplash. Journal of Musculoskeletal Pain 1993;1:89-131.

69. Jacome DE. Basilar artery migraine after uncomplicated whiplash injuries. Headache 1986;26:515-516.

70. Jacome DE. EEG in whiplash: a reappraisal. Clinical Electroencephography 1987;18:41-45.

71. Jensen MC, Brant-Zawadzki MN, Obuchowski N. Magnetic resonance imaging of the lumbar spine in people without back pain. New England Journal of Medicine 1994;331:69-73.

72. Katz RT. Carpal tunnel syndrome: a practical review. American Family Physician 1994;49;6;1371-1379.

73. Kellgren JH. Observations on referred pain arising from muscle. Clinical Science 1938;3:175-190.

74. Kelly RE. Post-traumatic syndrome. Journal of the Royal Society of Medicine 1981;74:242-244.

75. Kenna C, Murtagh J. Whiplash. Australian Family Physician 1987;16:727-736.

76. Khurana RK, Nirankari VS. Bilateral sympathetic dysfunction in post-traumatic headaches. Headache 1986;26:183-188.

77. Kidd RF, Nelson R. Musculoskeletal dysfunction of the neck in migraine and tension headache. Headache 1993;33:566-569.

78. Koes BW, Bouter LM, van Mameren H, Essers AHM et al. The effectiveness of manual therapy, physiotherapy, and treatment by the general practitioner for nonspecific back and neck complaints. Spine 1992;17:28.

79. Koes BW, Bouter LM, van Mameren H et al. Randomised clinical trial of manipulative therapy and physiotherapy for persistent back and neck compaints: results of one year follow up. BMJ 1992;304:601-605.

80. Kuch K, Swinson RP, Kirby M. Post-traumatic stress disorder after car accidents. Canadian Journal of Psychiatry 1985;30:426-7.

81. LaBan MM. "Whiplash": its evaluation and treatment. Physical Medicine and Rehabilitation 1990;4;2:293-307.

82. Lader F. Cervical trauma as a factor in the development of temporomandibular joint dysfunction and facial pain. Journal of Craniomandibular Practice 1983;1:86.

83. Ledingham J, Doherty S, Doherty M. Primary fibromyalgia syndrome — an outcome study. Br Journal of Rheumatology 1993;32:139-142.

84. Lee J, Giles K, Drummond P. Psychological disturbances and an exaggerated response to pain in patients with whiplash injury. Journal of Psychosomatic Research 1993;37:105-110.

85. Lehmann ECH. Accident neurosis: an orthopedic surgeon's view. BC Medical Journal 1991;33:657-661.

86. Levandoski RR. Mandibular whiplash, Part 1: an extension flexion injury of the temporomandibular joints. The Functional Orthodontist 1993;Jan/Feb:26-33.

87. Lindgren KA, Oksala I. Long-term outcome of surgery for thoracic outlet syndrome. American Journal of Surgery 1995;169:358-360.

88. Loebl S, Spratto GR, Woods AL. *The Nurse's Drug Handbook*, 1994.

89. Louis DS. Commentary: Progress? At what price? Journal of Hand Surgery 1995;20A:172.

90. Luo Z, Goldsmith W. Reaction of a human head/neck/torso system to shock. Journal of Biomechanics 1991;24;7;499-510.

91. MacNab I. Acceleration injuries of the cervical spine. Journal of Bone and Joint Surgery 1964;46A:1797-1799.

92. MacNab I. The whiplash syndrome. Orthopedic Clinics of North America 1971;2:389-403.

93. Maimaris C, Barnes MR, Allen MJ. 'Whiplash injuries' of the neck: a retrospective study. Injury 1988;19:393-6.

94. Matthews WB. Footballer's migraine. British Medical Journal 1972;2:326-327.

95. Mayou R, Bryant B, Duthie R. Psychiatric consequences of road traffic accidents. BMJ 1993;307:647-651.

96. Melzack R, Jeans ME, Stratford JG, Monks RC. Ice massage and transcutaneous electrical stimulation: comparison of treatment for low back pain. Pain 1980;9:209-217.

97. Mendelson G. Compensation, pain complaints, and psychological disturbance. Pain 1984;20:169-177.

98. Mendelson G. Not 'cured by a verdict': effect of legal settlement on compensation claimants. Medical Journal of Australia 1982;2:132-134.

99. Merskey H. Psychiatry and the cervical sprain syndrome. Canadian Medical Association Journal 1984;130:1119-1121.

100. Miller H. Accident neurosis. British Medical Journal 1961;1:919-925;992-998.

101. Moldofsky H, Wong MT, Lue FA. Litigation, sleep, symptoms and disabilities in postaccident pain (fibromyalgia). Journal of Rheumatology 1993;20:1935-40.

102. Muse M. Stress-related, posttraumatic chronic pain syndrome: behavioral treatment approach. Pain 1986;25:389-394.

103. Muse M. Stress-related, posttraumatic chronic pain syndrome: criteria for diagnosis, and preliminary report on prevalance. Pain 1985;23:295-300.

104. Mynors-Wallis LM, Gath DH, Lloyd-Thomas AR, Tomlinson D. Randomised controlled trial comparing problem solving treatment with amitriptyline and placebo for major depression in primary care. BMJ 1995;310:441-445.

105. Norris SH, Watt I. The prognosis of neck injuries resulting from rear-end vehicle collisions. Journal of Bone and Joint Surgery 1983;65B:608-611.

106. North RB, Campbell JN, James CS et al. Failed back surgery syndrome: 5-year follow-up in 102 patients undergoing repeated operation. Neurosurgery 1991;28:685-691.

107. Olson M, Sneed N. Anxiety and therapeutic touch. Issues in Mental Health Nursing 1995;16:97-108.

108. Ommaya AK, Yarnell P. Subdural hematoma after whiplash injury. The Lancet 1969;2:237-239.

109. Ommaya AK, Faas F, Yarnell P. Whiplash injury and brain damage — an experimental study. Journal of the American Medical Association 1968;204:285-289.

110. Osterweis M, Kleinman A, Mechanic D. Pain and disability: clinical, behavioral and public policy perspectives. Washington, DC, National Academy Press, 1987.

111. Packard RC, Ham LP. Posttraumatic headache. Journal of Neuropsychiatry 1994;6:229-236.

112. Parmar HV, Raymakers R. Neck injuries from rear impact road traffic accidents: prognosis in persons seeking compensation. Injury 1993;24:75-78.

113. Pearce JMS. Whiplash injury: a reappraisal. Journal of Neurology, Neurosurgery, and Psychiatry 1989;52:1329-1331.

114. Pearce JMS. Polemics of chronic whiplash injury. Neurology 1994;44:1993-1997.

115. Pettersson K, Hildingsson C, Toolanen G et al. MRI and neurology in acute whiplash trauma. Acta Orthopedica Scandinavica 1994;65:525-528.

116. Powers R. Fibromyalgia: an age-old malady begging for respect. Journal of General Internal Medicine 1993;8;93-105.

117. Press JM, Young JL. Vague upper-extremity symptoms? Consider thoracic outlet syndrome. Physical and Sports Medicine 1994;22:57-64.

118. Radanov BP, Di Stefano G, Schnidrig A, Ballinari P. Role of psychosocial stress in recovery from common whiplash. The Lancet 1991;338:712-715.

119. Radanov BP, Di Stefano G, Schnidrig A, Sturzenegger M. Common whiplash: psychosomatic or somatopsychic. Journal of Neurology, Neurosurgery, and Psychiatry 1994;57:486-490.

120. Radanov BP, Hirlinger I, Di Stefano G, Valach L. Attentional processing in cervical spine syndromes. Acta Neurologica Scandinavica 1992;85:358-362.

121. Radanov BP, Schnidrig A, Di Stefano G, Sturzenegger M. Illness behaviour after common whiplash. The Lancet 1992;339:749-750.

122. Radanov BP, Di Stefano G, Schnidrig A, Sturzenegger M. Psychosocial stress, congnitive performance and disability after common whiplash. Journal of Psychosomatic Research 1993;37:1-10.

123. Radanov BP, Sturzenegger M, Di Stefano G, Schnidrig A, Aljinovic M. Factors influencing recovery from headache after common whiplash. BMJ 1993;307:652-655.

124. Romano TJ. Clinical experiences with post-traumatic fibromyalgia syndrome. West Virginia Medical Journal 1990;86:198-202.

125. Roos DB, Owens JC. Thoracic outlet syndrome. Archives of Surgery 1966;93:71-74.

126. Roydhouse RH. Torquing of neck and jaw due to belt restraint in whiplash-type accidents. The Lancet 1985;June 8;p. 1341.

127. Sanders RJ. *Thoracic outlet syndrome: a common sequela of neck injuries*, 1991.

128. Sanders RJ, Pearce WH. The treatment of thoracic outlet syndrome: a comparison of different operations. Journal of Vascular Surgery 1989;10:626-634.

129. Schartz L, Slater MA, Birchler GR. Interpersonal stress and pain behaviors in patients with chronic pain. Journal of Consulting and Clinical Psychology 1994;62:861-864.

130. Schofferman J, Wasserman S. Successful treatment of low back pain and neck pain after a motor vehicle accident despite litigation. Spine 1994;19:1007-1010.

131. Schreiber S, Galai-Gat T. Uncontrolled pain following physical injury as the core trauma in post-traumatic stress disorder. Pain 1993;54:107-110.

132. Schutt CH, Dohan FC. Neck injury to women in auto accidents: a metropolitan plague. Journal of the American Medical Association 1968;206:2689-2692.

133. Selecki BR. Whiplash: a specialist's view. Australian Family Physician 1984;13:243-247.

134. Severy DM, Mathewson JH, Bechtol CO. Controlled automobile rear-end collisions, an investigation of related engineering and medical phenomena. Canadian Services Medical Journal 1955;11;727-759.

135. Shekelle PG, Adams AH, Chassin MR et al. Spinal manipulation for low back pain. Annals Internal Medicine 1992;117:590-598.

136. Smythe HA. The C6-7 syndrome — clinical features and treatment response. Journal of Rheumatology 1994;21;8:1520-6.

137. Sturzenegger M, DiStefano G, Radanov BP, Schnidrig A. Presenting symptoms and signs after whiplash injury: the influence of accident mechanisms. Neurology 1994;44:688-693.

138. Sucher BM. Thoracic outlet syndrome — a myofascial variant: part 1. Pathology and diagnosis. Journal of the American Osteopathic Association 1990;90:686-703.

139. Sucher BM. Myofascial manipulative release of carpal tunnel syndrome: documentation with magnetic resonance imaging. Journal of the American Osteopathic Association 1993;93:1273-1278.

140. Sucher BM. Myofascial release of carpal tunnel syndrome. Journal of the American Osteopathic Association 1993;93:92-101.

141. Sucher BM. Palpatory diagnosis and manipulative management of carpal tunnel syndrome. Journal of the American Osteopathic Association 1994;94;647-663.

142. Sucher BM. Thoracic outlet syndrome — a myofascial variant: part 2. Treatment. Journal of the American Osteopathic Association 1990;90:810-823.

143. Tamura T. Cranial symptoms after cervical injury. Aetiology and treatment of the Barre-Lieou syndrome. Journal of Bone and Joint Surgery 1989;71B:283-287.

144. Taylor VM, Deyo RA, Cherkin DC, Kreuter W. Low back pain hospitalization: recent United States trends and regional variations. Spine 1994;19:1207-1213.

145. Teasell RW, McCain GA. Clinical spectrum and management of whiplash injuries, in *Painful Cervical Trauma: Diagnosis and Rehabilitative Treatment of Neuromuscular Injuries*, Ed. Tollison CD, Satterthwaite JR 1992;292-318.

146. The Merck Manual of Diagnosis and Therapy, 1992

147. The Classic. Clinical Orthopedics and Related Research 1992;279:7

148. Torres F, Shapiro SK. Electroencephalograms in whiplash injury. Archives of Neurology 1961;5:28-35.

149. Valente R, Gibson H. Chiropractic manipulation in carpal tunnel syndrome. Journal of Manipulative and Physiological Therapeutics 1994;17;4;246-249.

150. van der Kolk BA, Dreyfuss D, Michaels M et al. Fluoxetine in posttraumatic stress disorder. Journal of Clinical Psychiatry 1994;55:517-522.

151. Waylonis GW, Perkins, RH. Post-traumatic fibromyalgia: a long-term follow-up. American Journal of Physical Medicine and Rehabilitation 1994;73:403-412.

152. Weinberg S, Lapointe H. Cervical extension-flexion injury (whiplash) and internal derangement of the temporomandibular joint. Journal of Oral and Maxillofacial Surgery 1987;45:653-656.

153. Weiss HD, Stern BJ, Goldberg J. Post-traumatic migraine: chronic migraine precipitated by minor head or neck trauma. Headache 1991;31:451-456.

154. Wiley AM et al. Musculoskeletal seequelae of whiplash injuries. Advocates Quarterly 1986;7:65-73.

155. Wolfe F, Smythe HA, Yunus MB et al. The American College of Rheumatology 1990 criteria for the classification of fibromyalgia. Arthritis & Rheumatism 1990;33:160-172.

156. Wolfe F, Cathey MA, Hawley DJ. A double-blind placebo controlled trial of fluoxetine in fibromyalgia. Scandanavian Journal of Rheumatology 1994;23:255-9.

157. Wolff's Headache and Other Head Pain, 1987. Edited by Dalessio DJ. Pp. 185-186.

158. Travell JG, Simons DG. Myofascial Pain and Dysfunction. The Trigger Point Manual. Baltimore, Williams & Wilkins, 1983.

159. Raskin NH. *Headache*, ed. 2. New York, Churchill Livingston Inc, 1988.

160. Vijayan N. A new post-traumatic headache syndrome. Headache 1977;17:19-22.

161. Hinoki M. Vertigo due to whiplash injury: a neurotological approach. Acta Otolaryngology (Stockh) 1985;419(suppl):9-29.

162. Greenfield J, Ilfeld FW. Acute cervical strain: evaluation and short term prognostic factors. Clinical Orthopedics 1977;122:196-200.

163. Mealy K, Brennan H, Fenelon GCC. Early mobilization of acute whiplash injuries. British Medical Journal 1986;292:656-657.

164. Anonymous. Neck injury and the mind. The Lancet 1991;338:728-729.

165. King AI. Point of view. Spine 1994;19:1290.

166. Packard RC. What does the headache patient want? Headache 1979;19:370-374.

167. Encel S, Johnston CE. Compensation and Rehabilitation. A survey of Worker's Compensation Cases Involving Back Injuries and Lump Sum Settlements, New South Wales University Press, Sydney, 1978.

168. Radanov BP, Sturzenegger M, De Stefano G. Long-term outcome after whiplash injury. A two-year follow-up considering the features of injury mechanisms and somatic, radiologic, and psychosocial findings. Medicine 1995;74(5):281-296.

169. Adler RH, Zamboni P, Hofer T, et al. How not to miss a somatic needle in the haystack of chronic pain. Journal of Psychosomatic Research 1997;42(5):499-506.

170. Agran P, Winn D, Dunkle D. Injuries among 4- to 9-year-old restrained motor vehicle occupants by seat location and crash impact site. American Journal of Disease in Childhood 1989;143:1317.

171. Aldman B. An analytical approach to the impact biomechanics of head and neck. Proceedings 30th Annual AAAM Conference 1986:439-454.

172. Amir M, Kaplan Z, Neumann L, Sharabani R, Shani N, and Buskila D. Posttraumatic stress disorder, tenderness, and fibromyalgia. Journal of Psychosomatic Research 1997;42(6):607-613

173. Andary MT, Crewe N, Ganzel SK, et al. Traumatic brain injury/chronic pain syndrome: a case comparison study. The Clinical Journal of Pain 1997;13:244-250.

174. Anisur Rahman MA, Jayson MIV, Black CM. Five patients who developed systemic sclerosis shortly after episodes of physical trauma. The Journal of Rheumatology 1996;23(10):1816-1817.

175. Anson J, Crowell RM. Cervicocranial arterial dissection. Neurosurgery 1991;29:89-96.

176. BenEliyahu DJ. Magnetic resonance imaging and clinical follow-up: study of 27 patients receiving chiropractic care for cervical and lumbar disc herniations. Journal of Manipulative and Physiological Therapeutics 1996;19(9):597-606.

177. Benito MC, Garcia F, Fernandez-Quero L, et al. Lesion of the internal carotid artery caused by a car safety belt. Journal of Trauma 1990;30(1):116-117.

178. Benzel EC, Hart BL, Ball PA, et al. Magnetic resonance imaging for the evaluation of patients with occult cervical spine injury. Journal of Neurosurgery 1996;85:824-829.

179. Wallis BJ, Lord SM, Barnsley L, Bogduk N.The psychological profiles of patients with whiplash-associated headache. Cephalgia 1998;18:101-105.

180. Bodack M, Tunkel R, et al. Spinal accessory nerve palsy as a cause of pain after whiplash injury: case report. Journal of Pain and Symptom Management 1998;15(5):321-328.

181. Boden SC. Point of View. Spine 1997;22(3):288.

182. Bogduk N. The anatomy of occipital neuralgia. Clinical and Experimental Neurology 1981;17:167-184.

183. Borchgrevink GE, Stiles TC, Borchgrevink PC, Lereim I. Personality profile among symptomatic and recovered patients with neck sprain injury, measured by MCMI-1 acutely and 6 months after car accidents. Journal of Psychosomatic Research 1997;42(4):357-367.

184. Borchgrevnick GE, Lereim I, Royneland L, et al. National health insurance consumption and chronic symptoms following mild neck sprain injuries in car collisions. Scandinavian Journal of Social Medicine 1996;24(4): 264-271.

185. Bostrom M. Summary of the Mayday Fund Survey: public attitudes about pain and analgesics. Journal of Pain and Symptom Management 1997;13(3):166-168.

186. Bourbeau R, Desjardins D, Maag U, Laberge-Nadeau C. Neck injuries among belted and unbelted occupants of the front seat of cars. The Journal of Trauma 1993;35(5):794-799.

187. Brault JR, Wheeler JB, Siegmund GP, Brault EJ. Clinical response of human subjects to rear-end automobile collisions. Archives of Physical Medicine and Rehabilitation 1998;79:72-80.

188. Braun BL, DiGiovanna A, Schiffman E, et al. A cross-sectional study of temporomandibular joint dysfunction in post-cervical trauma patients. Journal of Craniomandibular Disorders 1992;6(1):24-31.

189. Bu'Lock FA, Prothero A, Shaw C, et al. Cardiac involvement in seatbelt-related and direct sternal trauma: a prospective study and management implications. European Heart Journal 1994;15:1621-1627.

190. Buckley TC, Blanchard EB, Hickling EJ. A prospective examination of delayed onset PTSD secondary to motor vehicle accidents. Journal of Abnormal Psychology 1996;105(4):617-625.

191. Burgess JA, Dworkin SF. Litigation and post-traumatic TMD: how patients report treatment outcome. Journal of the American Dental Association 1993;124:105-110.

192. Burgess JA, Kolbinson DA, Lee PT, Epstein JB. Motor vehicle accidents and TMDS: assessing the relationship. Journal of the American Dental Association (JADA) 1996;127:1767-1772.

193. Buskila D, Neumann L, Vaisberg G, Alkalay D, Wolfe F. Increased rates of fibromyalgia following cervical spine injury: a controlled study of 161 cases of traumatic injury. Arthritis & Rheumatism 1997;40(3):446-452.

194. Bylund P, Bjornstig U. Sick leave and disability pension among passenger car occupants injured in urban traffic. Spine 1998; 23(9):1023-1028.

195. Carlier IVE, Lamberts RD, Van Uchelen AJ, et al. Clinical utility of a brief diagnostic test for posttraumatic stress disorder. Psychosomatic Medicine 1998;60:42-47.

196. Carr S, Troop B, Hurley J, et al. Blunt-trauma carotid artery injury: mild symptoms may disguise serious trouble. The Physician and Sportsmedicine 1996;24(2):48-54.

197. Chedid MK, Deeb ZL, Rothfus WE, et al. Major cerebral vessels injury caused by a seatbelt shoulder strap: case report. Journal of Trauma 1989;29(11):1601-1603.

198. Cholewicki J, Panjabi MM, Nibu K, Macius ME. Spinal ligament transducer based on a hall effect sensor. Journal of Biomechanics 1997;30(3):291-293.

199. Christensen LV, McKay DC. Reflex jaw motions and jaw stiffness pertaining to whiplash injury of the neck. Journal of Craniomandibular Practice 1997;15(3):242-260.

200. Christie B. Appeal overturns link between multiple sclerosis and whiplash. BMJ 1998;316:799.

201. Christie B. Multiple sclerosis linked to trauma in court case. BMJ 1996;313(7067):1228.

202. Cicerone KD, Kalmar K. Does premorbid depression influence post-concussive symptoms and neuropsychological functioning? Brain Injury 1997;11(9):643-648.

203. de Wijer A, de Leeuw RJ, Steenks MH, Bosman F. Temporomandibular and cervical spine disorders: self-reported signs and symptoms. Spine 1996;21(14):1638-1646.

204. Desfontaines Ph, Despland PA. Dissection of the internal carotid artery: aetiology, symptomatology, clinical and neuroonological follow-up, and treatment in 60 consecutive cases. Acta Neurologica Belgica 1995;95:226-234.

205. Di Gallo A, Barton J, Parry-Jones WL. Road traffic accidents: early psychological consequences in children and adolescents. British Journal of Psychiatry 1997;170:358-362.

206. DiPiro P, Meyer JE, Frenna TH, Denison CM. Seat belt injuries of the breast: findings on mammography and sonography. AJR 1995;164(Feb):317-320.

207. Dolinis J. Risk factors for 'whiplash' in drivers: a cohort study of rear-end traffic crashes. Injury 1997;28(3):173-179

208. Drottning M, Staff PH, Levin L, Malt UF. Acute emotional response to common whiplash predicts subsequent pain complaints—a prospective study of 107 subjects sustaining whiplash injury. Nord J Psychiat 1995;49:293-299.

209. Duckro PN, Chibnall JT, Greenberg MS, et al. Prevalence of temporomandibular dysfunction in chronic post-traumatic headache patients. Headache Quarterly 1997;8(3):228-233.

210. Ellis SJ. Tremor and other movement disorders after whiplash type injuries. Journal of Neurology, Neurosurgery, and Psychiatry 1997;63:110-112.

211. Epstein JB. Temporomandibular disorders, facial pain and headache following motor vehicle accidents. Scientific Journal 1992; 58:488-492.

212. Evans L, Gerrish PH. Antilock brakes and risk of front and rear impact in two-vehicle crashes. Accident Analysis and Prevention 1996;28(3):315-323.

213. Evans RW. Whiplash injuries. In: Macfarlane R, Hardy DG, eds. Outcome after head, neck and spinal trauma. Oxford, etc: Butterworth Heinemann, 1997:359-372.

214. Fattori B, Borsari C, Vannucci G, et al. Acupuncture treatment for balance disorders following whiplash injury. International Journal of Acupuncture and Electro-Therapeutics Research 1996;21:207-217.

215. Fisher CM. Concussion amnesia. Neurology 1966;16:826-830.

216. Fitzcharles MA, Esdaile JM. The overdiagnosis of fibromyalgia syndrome. American Journal of Medicine 1997;103:44-50.

217. Fitzgerald DC. Head trauma: hearing loss and dizziness. The Journal of Trauma: Injury, Infection, and Critical Care 1996;40(3):488-496.
218. Fredin Y, Elert J, Britschgi N, et al. A decreased ability to relax between repetitive muscle contractions in patients with chronic symptoms after whiplash trauma of the neck. Journal of Musculoskeletal Pain 1997;5(2):55-70.
219. Freeman MD, Croft AC, Rossignol AM. "Whiplash associated disorders: redefining whiplash and its management" by the Quebec Task Force: a critical evaluation. Spine 1998;23(9):1043-1049.
220. Fukui S, Ohseto K, Shiotani M et al. Referred pain distribution of the cervical zygapophysial joints and cervical dorsal rami. Pain 1996;68:79-83.
221. Galer BS, Schwartz L, Turner JA. Do patient and physician expectations predict response to pain-relieving procedures? The Clinical Journal of Pain 1997;13:348-351.
222. Garcia R, Arrington JA. The relationship between cervical whiplash and temporomandibular joint injuries: an MRI study. The Journal of Craniomandibular Practice 1996;14(3):233-239.
223. Garcia R. Airbag implicated in temporomandibular joint injury. Journal of Craniomandibular Practice 1994;12:125-127.
224. Gargan M, Bannister G, Main C, Hollis S. The behavioural response to whiplash injury. Journal of Bone and Joint Surgery [British] 1997;79-B:523-526.
225. Geisser ME, Roth RS, Bachman JE, Eckert TA. The relationship between symptoms of post-traumatic stress disorder and pain, affective disturbance and disability among patients with accident and non-accident related pain. Pain 1996;66:207-214.
226. Giacobetti FB, Vaccaro AR, Bos-Giacobetti MA, et al. Vertebral artery occlusion associated with cervical spine trauma. Spine 1997;22(2):188-192.
227. Gilkey SJ, Ramadan NM, Aurora TK, Welch KMA. Cerebral blood flow in chronic posttraumatic headache. Headache 1997;37:583-587.
228. Gimse R, Bjorgen IA, Staume A. Driving skills after whiplash. Scandinavian Journal of Psychology 1997;38(3):165-170.
229. Gimse R, Tjell C, Bjorgen IA, Saunte C. Disturbed eye movements after whiplash due to injuries to the posture control system. Journal of Clinical and Experimental Neuropsychology 1996;18(2):178-186.
230. Givens TG, Polley KA, Smith GF, Hardin WD. Pediatric cervical spine injury: a three-year experience. The Journal of Trauma: Injury, Infection, and Critical Care 1996;41(2):310-314.
231. Goldberg MB, Mock D, Ichise M, et al. Neuropsychologic deficits and clinical features of posstraumatic temporomandibular joint diosrders. Journal of Orofacial Pain 1996;10(2):126-140.
232. Grauer JN, Panjabi MM, Cholewicki J, Nibu K, Dvorak J. Whiplash produces an s-shaped curvature of the neck with hyperextension at lower levels. Spine 1997;22:2489-2494.
233. Greco CM, Rudy TE, Turk DC, Herlich A, Zaki HH. Traumatic onset of temporomandibular disorders: positive effects of a standardized conservative treatment program. The Clinical Journal of Pain 1997;13:337-347.
234. Griep EN, Boersma JW, Lentjes EG, et al. Function of the hypothalamic-pituitary-adrenal axis in patients with fibromyalgia and low back pain. The Journal of Rheumatology 1998;25:1374-1381.
235. Guertler AT. Blunt laryngeal trauma associated with shoulder harness use. Annals of Emergency Medicine 1988;17(8):838-839.
236. Hagström Y, Carlsson J. Prolonged functional impairments after whiplash injury. Scandinavian Journal of Rehabilitation Medicine 1996;28:139-146.
237. Harder S, Veilleuz M, Suissa S. The effect of socio-demographic and crash-related factors on the prognosis of whiplash. Journal of Clinical Epidemiology 1998; 51(5):377-384.
238. Hart RG, Easton JD. Dissection of cervical and vertebral arteries. Neurologic Clinics 1983;1:155-182.
239. Hartmann PK, Mintz G, Verne D, et al. Diagnosis and primary management of laryngeal trauma. Oral Surgery Oral Medicine and Oral Pathology 1985;60:252-257.
240. Heikkilä H, Åström PG. Cervicocephalic kinesthetic sensibility in patients with whiplash injury. Scandinavian Journal of Rehabilitation Medicine 1996;28:133-138.

241. Hendler N, Bergson C, Morrison C. Overlooked physical diagnosis in chronic pain patients involved in litigation, part 2: the addition of MRI, nerve blocks, 3-D CT, and Qualitative Flow Meter. Psychosomatics 1996; 37(6):509-517.

242. Hobson DE, Gladish DF. Botulinum toxin injection for cervicogenic headache. Headache 1997;37:253-255.

243. Hodge JR. The whiplash neurosis. Psychosomatics 1971;12:245-249.

244. Huelke DF, Moore JL, Compton TW, et al. Upper extremity injuries related to airbag deployments. The Journal of Trauma 1995;38(4):482-488.

245. Hurwitz EL, Aker PD, Adams AH, et al. Manipulation and mobilization of the cervical spine: a systematic review of the literature. Spine 1996;21(15):1746-1760.

246. Huston BL, King TP. An analytical assessment of three point restraints in several accident configurations. Paper presented to Automatic Occupant Protection Systems, International Congress and Exposition, Detroit, Michigan, February 29-March 4, 1988, pp. 55-59.

247. Insurance Institute for Highway Safety, Status Report, Special Issue: Whiplash Injuries. September 16, 1995.

248. Janhangir Janjua K, Goswami V, Sagar G. Whiplash injury associated with acute bilateral internal carotid artery dissection. The Journal of Trauma, Injury, Infection, and Critical Care 1996;40(2):456-458.

249. Jankovic J. Post-traumatic movement disorders: central and peripheral mechanisms. Neurology 1994;44:2006-14.

250. Kant R, Smith-Seemiller L, Isaac G, Duffy J. Tc-HMPAO SPECT in persistent post-concussion syndrome after mild head injury: comparison with MRI/CT. Brain Injury 1997;11(2):115-124.

251. Karlsborg M, Smed A, Jespersen H, et al. A prospective study of 39 patients with whiplash injury. Acta Neurologica Scandinavica 1997;95:65-72.

252. Kelly JP, Rosenberg JH. Diagnosis and management of concussion in sports. Neurology 1997;48:575-580.

253. Kessels RPC, Keyser A, Verhagen WIM, et al. The whiplash syndrome: a psychophysiological and neuropsychological study towards attention. Acta Neurologica Scandinavica 1998;97:188-193.

254. Klimczak NJ, Donovick PJ, Burright R. The malingering of multiple sclerosis and mild traumatic brain injury. Brain Injury 1997;11(5):343-352.

255. Kolbinson DA, Epstein JB, Burgess JA, Senthilselvan A. Temporomandibular disorders, headaches, and neck pain after motor vehicle accidents: a pilot investigation of persistence and litigation effects. The Journal of Prosthetic Dentistry 1997;77(1):46-53.

256. Kolbinson DA, Epstein JB, Senthilselvan A, Burgess JA. A comparison of TMD patients with or without prior motor vehicle accident involvement: treatment and outcomes. Journal of Orofacial Pain 1997;11:337-345.

257. Kolbinson DA, Epstein JB, Senthilselvan A, Burgess JA. Effect of impact and injury characteristics on post-motor vehicle accident temporomandibular disorders. Oral surgery, Oral Medicine, Oral Pathology 1998; 85(6):665-673.

258. Kouyanou K, Pither C, Rabe-Haketh S, Wessely S. A comparative study of iatrogenesis, medication abuse, and psychiatric morbidity in chronic pain patients with and without medically explained symptoms. Pain 1998; 76: 417-426.

259. Kouyanou K, Pither CE, Wessely S. Iatrogenic factors and chronic pain. Psychosomatic Medicine 1997;59:597-604.

260. Kronn F. The incidence of TMJ dysfunction in patients who have suffered a cervical whiplash injury following a traffic accident. Journal of Orofacial Pain 1993;7(2):209-213.

261. Landy PJB. Neurological sequelae of minor head and neck injuries. Injury 1998;29(3):199-206.

262. Landy SH, Donovan TB, Laster RE. Repeat CT or MRI in posttraumatic headache. Headache 1996;36:44-47.

263. Larsson LG, Baum J, Muholkar GS. Hypermobility: features and differential incidence between the sexes. Arthritis & Rheumatism 1987;30:1426-1430.

264. Law Commission. Personal Injury Compensation: How Much is Enough? A Study of the Compensation Experiences of Victims of Personal Injury. 1994, London: HMSO.

265. Leckie RG, Buckner AB, Bornemann M. Seat belt-related thyroiditis documented with thyroid Tc-99m pertechnate scans. Clinical Nuclear Medicine 1992;17(Nov):859-860.

266. Lemmerling M, Crevits L, Defreyne L, et al. Traumatic dissection of the internal carotid artery as unusual cause of hypoglossal nerve dysfunction. Clinical Neurology and Neurosurgery 1996;98:52-54.

267. *Letters. The Lancet 1996;348:124-126.*

268. Lindgren KA. Conservative treatment of thoracic outlet syndrome: a 2-year follow-up. Archives of Physical Medicine and Rehabilitation 1997;78:373-378.

269. Lord SM, Barnsley L, Wallis BJ, Bogduk N. Chronic cervical zygapophysial joint pain after whiplash: a placebo-controlled prevalence study. Spine 1996;21(15):1737-1745.

270. Lord SM, Barnsley L, Wallis BJ, et al. Chronic cervical zygapophysial joint pain after whiplash. Spine 1996;21(15):1737-1745.

271. Lord SM, Barnsley L, Wallis BJ, et al. Percutaneous radio-frequency neurotomy for chronic cervical zygapophysial joint pain. New England Journal of Medicine 1996;335(23):1721-1726.

272. Loudon JK, Ruhl M, Field E. Ability to reproduce head position after whiplash injury. Spine 1997;22(8):865-868.

273. Lu J, Ebraheim NA. Anatomic considerations of C2 nerve root ganglion. Spine 1998;23(6):649-652.

274. Lundell B, Jakobsson L, Alfredsson B, Jernstrom C. Guidelines for and the design of a car seat concept for improved protection against neck injuries in rear end car impacts. Society of Automotive Engineers 1998; SAE 980301.

275. Lynch JM, Meza MP, Pollack IF, Adelson PD. Direct injury to the cervical spine of a child by a lap-shoulder belt resulting in quadraplegia: case report. The Journal of Trauma 1996;41(4):747-749.

276. Machulda MM, Bergquist TF, Ito V, Chew S. Relationship between stress, coping, and postconcussion symptoms in a healthy adult population. Archives of Clinical Neuropsychology 1998;13(5):415-424.

277. Magnusson T, Ragnarsson T, Bjornsson A. Occipital nerve release in patients with whiplash trauma and occipital neuralgia. Headache 1996;36:32-36.

278. Mailis A, Papagapiou M, Vanderlinden RG, et al. Thoracic outlet syndrome after motor vehicle accidents in a Canadian pain clinic population. The Clinical Journal of Pain 1995;11:316-324.

279. Mallinson AI, Longridge NS, Peacock C. Dizziness, imbalance, and whiplash. Journal of Musculoskeletal Pain 1996;4(4):105-112.

280. Malt UF, Olafsen OM. Psychological appraisal and emotional response to physical injury: a clinical, phenomenological study of 109 adults. Psychiatric Medicine 1992;10(3):117-0134.

281. Marchiori DM, Henderson CNR. A cross-sectional study correlating cervical radiographic degenerative findings to pain and disability. Spine 1996;21(23):2747-2752.

282. Martini G, Martini M, Carano A. MRI study of a physiotherapeutic protocol in anterior disk displacement without reduction. The Journal of Craniomandibular Practice 1996;14(3):216-224.

283. Mason LW, Goolkasian P, and McCain GA. Evaluation of a multimodal treatment program for fibromyalgia. Journal of Behavioral Medicine 1998;21(2):163-178.

284. Matsumoto M, Fujimara Y, Suzuki N, Ono T, et al. Relationship between cervical curvature and disc degeneration in asymptomatic subjects. Journal of Eastern Japan Association of Orthopaedics and Traumatology 1977;9:1-4.

285. Mayou R, Bryant B. Outcome of 'whiplash' neck injury. Injury 1996;27(9):617-623.

286. Mayou R, Tyndel S, Bryant B. Long-term outcome of motor vehicle accident injury. Psychosomatic Medicine 1997;59:578-584.

287. Mayou R. Accident neurosis revisited. British Journal of Psychiatry 1996;168:399-403.

288. McClelland RJ. The postconcussional syndrome: a rose by any other name. Journal of Psychosomatic Research 1996;40(6):563-568.

289. McConnell WE, Howard RP, Guzman HM, et al. Analysis of human test subject kinematic responses to low velocity rear end impacts. Society of Automotive Engineers 1993;SAE 930889.

290. McConnell WE, Howard RP, Van Poppel J, et al. Human head and neck kinematics after low-velocity rear-end impacts: understanding whiplash. Society of Automotive Engineers, SAE 952724.

291. McDermid AJ, Rollman GB, McCain GA. Generalized hypervigilance in fibromyalgia: evidence of perceptual amplification. Pain 1996;66:133-144.

292. Moore KL. Trauma and headaches. Headache Quarterly 1996;7(1):21-29.

293. Moore M. Thoracic outlet syndrome experience in a metropolitan hospital. Clinical Orthopedics 1986;207:29-30.

294. Moss NEG, Wade DT. Admission after head injury: how many occur and how many are recorded? Injury 1996;27(3):159-161.

295. Murray PA, Pitcher M, Galasko CSB. The cost of long-term disability from road traffic accidents: four year study: final report. Transport Research Laboratory. University of Manchester, 1993.

296. National Traffic Safety Administration: Air bag deployment characteristics. Springfield, Va, National Technical Information Service, September 1992.

297. Nibu K, Cholewicki J, Panjabi MM, Babat LB, et al. Dynamic elongation of the vertebral artery during an in vitro whiplash simulation. European Spine Journal 1997;6(4):286-289.

298. Nicassio PM, Radojevic V, Weisman MH, et al. A comparison of behavioral and educational interventions for fibromyalgia. Journal of Rheumatology 1997;24:2000-2007.

299. Ommaya AK, Gennarelli TA. Cerebral concussion and traumatic unconsciousness. Correlation of experimental and clinical observations on blunt head injuries. Brain 1974;97:633-654.

300. Ono K, Kaneoka K, Wittek A, Kajzer J. Cervical injury mechanism based on the analysis of human cervical vertebral motion and head-neck-torso kinematics during low speed rear impacts. Society of Automotive Engineers, 41st STAPP Car Crash Conference Proceedings 1997; SAE 973340.

301. Ortengren T, Hansson HA, Lovsund P, et al. Membrane leakage in spinal ganglion nerve cells induced by experimental whiplash extension motion: a study in pigs. Journal of Neurotrauma 1996;13(3):171-180.

302. Osberg JS, DiScala C. Morbidity among pediatric motor vehicle crash victims: the effectiveness of seat belts. American Journal of Public Health 1992;823:422.

303. Otte A, Ettlin TM, Nitzsche EU, et al. PET and SPECT in whiplash syndrome: a new approach to a forgotten brain? Journal of Neurology, Neurosurgery, and Psychiatry 1997;63:368-372.

304. Otte A, Goetze M, Mueller-Brand J. Statistical parametric mapping in whiplash brain: is it only a contusion mechanism? European Journal of Nuclear Medicine [Letter] 1998;25:306-312.

305. Otte A, Mueller-Brand J, Fierz L. Brain SPECT findings in late whiplash syndrome. The Lancet, June 10, 1995;345:1513-1514.

306. Packard RC, Ham LP. Evaluation of cognitive evoked potentials in post-traumatic headache cases with cognitive dysfunction. Headache Quarterly, Current Treatment and Research 1996;7(3):218-224.

307. Parker RS, Rosenblum A. IQ loss and emotional dysfunctions after mild head injury incurred in a motor vehicle accident. Journal of Clinical Psychology 1996;52(1):32-43.

308. Parker RS. The spectrum of emotional distress and personality changes after minor head injury incurred in a motor vehicle accident. Brain Injury 1996;4:287-302.

309. Pearce JMS. Longus cervicis colli "myositis" (syn: retropharyngeal tendinitis). Journal of Neurology, Neurosurgery, and Psychiatry 1996;61:324.

310. Perlis M, Artiola L, Giles DE. Sleep complaints in chronic postconcussion syndrome. Perceptual and Motor Skills 1997; 84:595-599.

311. Pettersson K, Hildingsson C, Toolanen G, et al. Disc pathology after whiplash injury: a prospective magnetic resonance imaging and clinical investigation. Spine 1997;22(3):283-288.

312. Pettersson K, Toolanen G. High-dose methylprednisolone prevents extensive sick leave after whiplash injury. Spine 1998;23(9):984-989.

313. Poletti CE. Third cervical nerve root and ganglion compression: clinical syndrome, surgical anatomy, and pathological findings. Neurosurgery 1996;39(5):941-949.

314. Povlishock JT, Lontos HA. Continuing axonal and vascular change following experimental brain trauma. Journal of the Central Nervous System Trauma 1985;2:285-298.

315. Pritchett JW. C-reactive protein levels determine the severity of soft-tissue injuries. The American Journal of Orthopedics 1996;Nov:759-761.

316. Provinciali L, Baroni M, Illuminati L, Ceravolo MG. Multimodal treatment to prevent the late whiplash syndrome. Scandinavian Journal of Rehabilitation Medicine 1996;28:105-111.

317. Pullinger AG, Monteiro AA. History factors associated with symptoms of temporomandibular disorders. Journal of Oral Rehabilitation 1988;16:117-124.

318. Radanov BP, Begres, Sturzenegger M, Augustiny KF. Course of psychological variables in whiplash injury—a 2-year follow-up with age, gender and education pair-matched patients. Pain 1996;64:429-434.

319. Rapoport A, Stang P, Gutterman DL, et al. Analgesic rebound headache in clinical practice: data from a physician survey. Headache 1996;36:14-19.

320. Ratliff AHC. Whiplash injuries. [Editorial] Journal of Bone and Joint Surgery [British] 1997;79-B:517-519.

321. Reddy K, Furer M, West M, et al. Carotid artery dissection secondary to seatbelt trauma: case report. Journal of Trauma 1990;30(5):630-633.

322. Report of the Ad Hoc Committee to Study Head Injury Nomenclature. Proceedings of the Congress of Neurological Surgeons in 1964. Clinical Neurosurgery 1966;12:386-394.

323. Restifo KM, Kelen GD. Case report: sternal fracture from a seatbelt. The Journal of Emergency Medicine 1994;12(3):321-323.

324. Robbins MC. Lack of relationship between vehicle damage and occupant injury. SAE 970494

325. Rogers RG. The effects of spinal manipulation on cervical kinesthesia in patients with chronic neck pain: a pilot study. Journal of Manipulative and Physiological Therapeutics 1997;20(2):80-85.

326. Rosenhall U, Johansson G, Orndahl G. Otoneurologic and audiologic findings in fibromyalgia. Scandinavian Journal of Rehabilitation Medicine 1996;28:225-232.

327. Roydhouse RH. Whiplash and temporomandibular joint dysfunction. Lancet 1973;1:394.

328. Rubin AM, Woolley SM, Dailey VM, Goebel JA. Postural stability following mild head or whiplash injuries. The American Journal of Otology 1995;16(2):216-221.

329. Ruff RM, Camenzuli L, Mueller J. Miserable minority: emotional risk factors that influence the outcome of a mild traumatic brain injury. Brain Injury 1996;10(8):551-565.

330. Rupprecht H, Rumenapf G, Braig H, Flesch R. Acute bleeding caused by rupture of the thyroid gland following blunt neck trauma: case report. Journal of Trauma 1994;36(3):408-409.

331. Saal JS, Saal JA, Yurth EF. Nonoperative management of herniated cervical intervertebral disc with radiculopathy. Spine 1996;21(16):1877-1883.

332. Sastry SM, Copeland RA, Mezghebe H, Siram SM. Retinal hemorrhage secondary airbag-related ocular trauma. The Journal of Trauma 1995;38(4):582.

333. Satoh S, Naito S, Konishi T, et al. An examination of reasons for prolonged treatment in Japanese patients with whiplash injuries. Journal of Musculoskeletal Pain 1997;5(2):71-84.

334. Savolaine ER, Ebraheim NA, Hoeflinger M, et al. Subluxation of the cervical spine caused by 3-point seat belt. Orthopedic Review 1994;235:439.

335. Schmand B, Lindeboom J, Schagen S, et al. Cognitive complaints in patients after whiplash injury: the impact of malingering. Journal of Neurology, Neurosurgery and Psychiatry 1998;64:339-343

336. Schrader H, Obelieniene D, Bovim G, et al. The Lancet 1996;347:1207-1211.

337. Smed A. Cognitive function and distress after common whiplash injury. Acta Neurologica Scandinavica 1997;95:73-80.

338. Spafford Smock W, Nichols GR. Airbag module cover injuries. The Journal of Trauma 1995;38(4):489-493.

339. Special Issue: Head restraints. Insurance Institute for Highway Safety. Status Report 1997;32(4).

340. Spitzer WO, Skovron ML, Salmi LR, et al. Scientific monograph of the Quebec task force on whiplash-associated disorders: Redefining 'whiplash' and its management. Spine 1995;20(suppl 8):1-73.

341. Squires B, Gargan MF, Bannister GC. Soft-tissue injuries of the cervical spine: 15-year follow-up. The Journal of Bone and Joint Surgery 1996;78-B(6):955-957.

342. Steigerwald DP, Verne SV, Young DN. A retrospective evaluation of the impact of temporomandibular joint arthroscopy on the symptoms of headache, neck pain, shoulder pain, dizziness, and tinnitus. CRANIO 1996;14(1):46-54.

343. Steuart RD, Morrison RT. Fracture of the laryngeal cartilage: an incidental finding on bone scintigraphy. Clinical Nuclear Medicine 1992;17(Oct):815-817.

344. Sunderland S. Nerves and Nerve Injuries 1978, Churchill Livingstone: Edinburgh.

345. Swartzman LC, Teasell RW, Shapiro AP, McDermid AJ. The effect of litigation status on adjustment to whiplash injury. Spine 1996;21(1):53-58.

346. Taylor AE, Cox CA, Mailis A. Persistent neuropsychological deficits following whiplash: evidence for chronic mild traumatic brain injury? Archives of Physical Medicine and Rehabilitation 1996;77(6):529-535.

347. Temming J. Human factors data in relation to whiplash injuries in rear end collisions of passenger cars. Society of Automotive Engineers 1998; SAE 981191.

348. Tennyson SA, King AI. A biodynamic model of the human spinal column. Proceedings of the SAE Mathematical Modeling Biodynamic Response to Impact. Society of Automotive Engineers, 31-44, 1976.

349. The Statesman's Year-Book, Statistical and historical annual of the states of the world for the year 1995-1996, ed. Brian Hunter. St. Martin's Press, New York: p. 887.

350. Tjell C, Rosenhall U. Smooth pursuit neck torsion test: a specific test for cervical dizziness. The American Journal of Otology 1998;19:76-81.

351. Turk DC, Okifuji A, Starz TW, Sinclair JD. Effects of symptom onset on psychological distress and disability in fibromyalgia syndrome patients. Pain 1996;68:423-430.

352. Van Goetham JWM, Biltjes IGGM, van den Hauwe L, et al. Whiplash injuries: is there a role for imaging? European Journal of Radiology 1996;22:30-37.

353. Viano DC, Gargan MF. Headrest position during normal driving: implication to neck injury risk in rear crashes. Accident Analysis and Prevention 1996;28(6):665-674.

354. Viktrup L, Knudsen GM, Hansen SH. Delayed onset of fatal basilar thrombotic embolus after whiplash injury. Stroke 1995;26(11):2194-2196.

355. Volans AP. The risks of minor head injury in the warfarinised patient. Journal of Accident Emergency Medicine 1998;15:159-161.

356. Von Korff M, Simon G. The relationship between pain and depression. British Journal of Psychiatry 1996;168(suppl 30):101-108.

357. Wachter KC, Kaeser HE, Guhring H, et al. Muscle damping measured with a modified pendulum test with patients fibromyalgia, lumbago, and cervical syndrome. Spine 1996;21(18):2137-2142.

358. Wallis BJ, Bogduk N. Faking a profile: can naïve subjects simulate whiplash responses? Pain 1996;66:223-227.

359. Wallis BJ, Lord SM, Barnsley L, Bogduk N. Pain and psychologic symptoms of Australian patients with whiplash. Spine 1996;21(7):804-810.

360. Wallis BJ, Lord SM, Bogduk N. Resolution of psychological distress of whiplash patients following treatment by radiofrequency neurotomy: a randomised, double-blind, placebo-controlled trial. Pain 1997;73:15-22.

361. Waterloo K, Ingebrigtsen T, Romner B. Neuropsychological function in patients with increased serum levels of protein S-100 after minor head injury. Acta Neurochirurgica 1997;139:26-32.

362. Westmark RM, Westmark KD, Sonntag VKH. Disappearing cervical disc: case report. Journal of Neurosurgery 1997;86:289-290.

363. Whiplash Injuries, Status Report, Insurance Institute for Highway Safety 1995;30(8) September 16, 1995.

364. Wiklund K, Larsson H. Saab active head restraint (SAHR)—seat design to reduce the risk of neck injuries in rear impacts. Society of Automotive Engineers 1998;SAE 980297.

365. Wolfe F, Anderson J, Harkness D, et al. The work and disability status of persons with fibromyalgia. Journal of Rheumatology 1997;24:1171-1178.

366. Wolfe F. The fibromyalgia problem. Editorial. Journal of Rheumatology 1997;24:1247-1249.

367. Wood KB, Garvey TA, Gundry C, et al. Magnetic resonance imaging of the thoracic spine: evaluation of asymptomatic individuals. The Journal of Bone and Joint Surgery November, 1995;77A(11):1631-1638.

368. Woodring JH, Lee C. Limitations of cervical radiography in the evaluation of acute cervical trauma. Journal of Trauma 1993;34:32-39.

369. Woodring JH, Lee C. The role and limitations of computed tomography scanning in the evaluation of cervical trauma. Journal of Trauma 1992;33:698-708.

370. Woodward MN, Cook JCH, Gargan MF, Bannister GC. Chiropractic treatment of chronic 'whiplash' injuries. Injury: International Journal of the Care of the Injured 1996;27(9):643-645.

371. Woolf CJ, Shortland P, Coggeshall RE. Peripheral nerve injury triggers central sprouting of myelinated afferents. Nature 1992;355:75.

372. Yang KH, Begeman PC, Muser M, et al. On the role of cervical facet joints in rear end impact neck injury mechanisms. Society of Automotive Engineers 1997;SAE 970497.

373. Yarnell R, Rossie GV. Minor whiplash head injury with major debilitation. Brain Injury 1988;3:255-258.

374. Otte A, Ettlin T, Fierz L, Mueller-Brand J. Parieto-occipital hypoperfusion in late whiplash syndrome: first quantitative SPET study using technetium-99m bicisate (ECD). European Journal of Nuclear Medicine 1996;23(1):72-74.

375. Kolbinson DA, Epstein JB, Burgess JA. Temporomandibular disorders, headaches, and neck pain following motor vehicle accidents and the effect of litigation: review of the literature. Journal of Orofacial Pain 1996;10:101-125.

376. Nielsen GP, Gough JP, Little DM, West DH, Baker VT. Human subject responses to repeated low speed impacts using utility vehicles. Society of Automotive Engineers 1997;SAE 970394.

377. Aaron LA, Bradley LA, Alarcon GS, et al. Perceived physical and emotional trauma as precipitating events in fibromyalgia. Arthritis & Rheumatism 1997;40(3):453-460.

378. Sjaastad O, Fredriksen TA, Pfaffenrath V. Cervicogenic headache: diagnostic criteria. Headache 1998;38:442-445.

379. Bryant RA, Harvey AG. Relationship between acute stress disorder and posttraumatic stress disorder following mild traumatic brain injury. American Journal of Psychiatry 1998;155(5):625-629.

380. Shalev AY, Freedman S, Peri T, et al. Prospective study of posttraumatic stress disorder and depression following trauma. American Journal of Psychiatry 1998;155(5):630-637.

381. Donaldson CCS, Nelson DV, Skubick DL, Clasby RG. Potential contributions of neck muscle dysfunctions to initiation and maintenance of carpal tunnel syndrome. Applied Psychophysiology and Biofeedback 1998;23(1):59-72.

382. Donaldson CCS, Nelson DV, Schulz R. Disinhibition in the gamma motoneuron circuitry: a neglected mechanism for understanding myofascial pain syndromes? Applied Psychophysiology and Biofeedback 1998;23(1):43-57.

383. Silver JM, McAllister TW. Forensic issues in the neuropsychiatric evaluation of the patient with mild traumatic brain injury. Journal of Neuropsychiatry 1997;9(1):102-113.

384. Evans RW. Whiplash Injuries, Chapter 25. Neurology and Trauma, edited by RW Evans. WB Saunders Company, 1996;39-457.

385. Szabo TJ, Welcher JB. Human subject kinematics and electromyographic activity during low speed rear impacts. 40th Stapp Car Crash Conference, SAE 962432.

386. Matsushita T, Sato TB, Hirabayashi K, et al. X-ray study of the human neck motion due to head inertia loading. 38th Stapp Car Crash Conference 1994; SAE 942208.

387. Inbody SB. Myofascial Pain Syndromes, In Neurology and Trauma, edited by Evans RW, W.B. Saunders Company 1996, p. 464.

388. Erichsen JE. Concussion of the Spine: Nervous Shock and other obscure injuries of the nervous system in their clinical and medico-legal aspects. William Wood and Co, New York. 1882.

389. Vernon H. The neck disability index: patient assessment and outcome monitoring in whiplash. Journal of Musculoskeletal Pain 1996;4(4):95-104.

Index